CBITS:
Cognitive Behavioral Intervention for Trauma in Schools

Lisa Jaycox, Ph.D.

ISBN 1-57035-975-X

Printed in the United States of America

Published and Distributed by

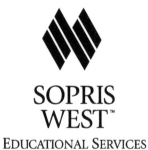

SOPRIS
WEST™
EDUCATIONAL SERVICES

A Cambium Learning™ Company

4093 Specialty Place • Longmont, CO 80504 • (303) 651-2829

www.sopriswest.com

62674/228CBITS/08-16

ACKNOWLEDGMENTS

Many people have contributed to the development and evaluation of this manual, which was funded by RAND Health and by the Los Angeles Unified School District (LAUSD) (Office of Student Intervention Services, Emergency Immigrant Education Program, and Mental Health Services). The investment in this work by Marleen Wong, Robert Barner, Lila Silvern, and Trude Skolnick at LAUSD made this work possible. Many thanks to my collaborators, Sheryl Kataoka, Bradley Stein, Marleen Wong, Arlene Fink, and Ken Wells, who provided valuable comments about this manual and its evaluation. Stephanie Cramer helped to conduct the first pilot test of this program, with the support of the UCLA/RAND Research Center on Managed Care for Psychiatric Disorders and RAND Health. Most of all, thanks to the clinicians who helped me refine the manual over three years with many helpful suggestions and revisions: Verenisa Alfaro, Erika Cedillos, Flor Chaidez, Christina Kim, Debora Presser, Lilliam E. Rodriguez, Deyanira Vera, Svetlana Vilsker, Anita Yousoofian, and Rosana Zatarain-Oyola, with support from Catalina Zaragoza, Pia Escudero, Cecilia Ramos, Michelle Rosemond, Carol McCauliffe, and Narod Simciyan.

I would like to acknowledge that the concepts and techniques presented in this program reflect the work of many esteemed clinicians and colleagues over the years, including Joan Asarnow, David Clark, Gregory Clarke, Constance Dancu, Jane Gillham, Diana Hearst-Ikeda, Elizabeth Hembree, Edna Foa, Elizabeth Meadows, Jeanne Miranda, Ricardo Munoz, Karen Reivich, and Martin E. P. Seligman. Some parts of this manual were derived from treatment manuals for other populations, and this manual would not have been possible without the years of work that developed those manuals and evaluated their efficacy. Where our exercises are derived from earlier or concurrent work, we note the relevant source so that interested group leaders may access those manuals and books.

The original source and rights owner of this manual is The RAND Corporation, Inc, a nonprofit research organization providing objective analysis and effective solutions that address the challenges facing the public and private sectors around the world.

ABOUT THE AUTHOR

Lisa Jaycox, Ph.D. is a behavioral scientist at RAND (Arlington, VA) and a clinical psychologist (University of Pennsylvania, 1993). Dr. Jaycox has combined clinical and research expertise in the areas of child and adolescent mental health problems, especially related to depression and reactions to violence exposure such as post-traumatic stress disorder. Jaycox developed and evaluated a school-based depression prevention program that proved to be effective in preventing the onset of severe depressive symptoms among fifth and sixth graders. She also evaluated psychosocial treatment and prevention of post-traumatic stress disorder among adult female assault survivors. Dr. Jaycox joined RAND in 1997 and is working on projects related to the treatment of adolescent depression in primary care settings, mental health consequences of community violence among young adults, evaluation of adolescent substance abuse treatment programs, use of trauma-focused therapy to improve school-based mental health services for children, and evaluation of an intimate partner violence prevention program for Latino youth.

CONTENTS

FOREWORD

It is an honor to welcome you to the *CBITS (Cognitive-Behavioral Intervention for Trauma in Schools)* program and to thank you for your commitment to providing evidenced-based interventions to children who have been exposed to violence.

In the wake of terrorist attacks in the U.S. and abroad, mental health professionals have become more aware than ever of the destructive effects of fear and violence on the lives of children. But even prior to September 11, 2001, school-based mental health professionals (including school counselors, school psychologists, and school social workers) were faced with the challenge of helping students who have been traumatized by violence in their homes, their schools, and their communities.

Public health officials have identified violence as one of the most significant public health issues facing America. Dr. Bradley Stein of The RAND Corporation, Inc writes, " . . . for many (children), personally experiencing or directly witnessing multiple incidents of community violence is the norm . . . the majority of youth exposed to community violence display post-traumatic stress symptoms, with a substantial minority developing clinically significant Post-traumatic Stress Disorder (PTSD)" (Stein et al., 2003).

Despite what we know about the disruptive and distressing symptoms of post-traumatic stress, PTSD, depression, and anxiety, we are not meeting the needs of children who suffer from the negative consequences of exposure to violence. There is so much we need to learn in order to bring more science to practice, especially in the practice of mental health in schools.

CBITS fills that vacuum. As reported in the *Journal of the American Medical Association*, this program for youth with symptoms resulting from violence exposure was shown in a randomized controlled study to be effective (Stein et al., 2003). Further, it has achieved this distinction in the context of providing services in real schools.

My enthusiasm for this work comes from many sources. As the former director of mental health services for the Los Angeles Unified School District, I saw my staff members build professional skills and deepen their understanding of the impact of violence on the social, behavioral, and academic lives of students. In my personal life, I've been a school board member, the daughter of an immigrant, a single parent, and a member of an ethnic minority whose first language was Cantonese.

From the time I was six years old, my grandmother told me stories about her early life in San Francisco. That beautiful city was part of the Wild West in the early 1900s, and for Chinese immigrants it was a vibrant and dangerous place. The residents of Chinatown were vulnerable to violence from both fellow residents, marauding gangs who victimized the restaurants and businesses (including "benevolent associations" known as Tongs who were waging a war for power in Chinatown), and from white criminals. Often, innocent people were caught in the crossfire. The process of immigration from Macao to San Francisco was no less dangerous. Pirates and thieves preyed on children and adults who boarded boats to escape the Boxer Rebellion in South China on their way to "Gold Mountain," the name that was given to California and the promises it held for a new life.

My grandmother was five when she took the long trip from Macao to San Francisco. As a child, she was terrified by the violence in the streets and businesses of Chinatown. Once, she saw a group of men refuse to pay their bill for dinner and many bottles of liquor. When the owner insisted, they drew guns and shot bullets into the walls and the floors, smashing the furniture and laughing as they left. She hid in a corner, unharmed but traumatized. In the following weeks, she refused to go to school or to leave her home. She feared that she would be killed and that the violence would happen again.

In 1905, there was no counseling available in schools nor was there recognition of the paralyzing effects of violence on children. The year my grandmother died, in 1999, I began my association with *CBITS* and, since that time, I've had the privilege of working with Dr. Jaycox. I have witnessed firsthand the transformation of children's lives. We have seen statistically significant reductions in the most serious symptoms of post-traumatic stress disorder, anxiety, and depression (Stein et al., 2003). We have also seen promising trends in improved academic performance and school attendance by the end of the school year.

The scars of violence can last a lifetime, but with early identification and early intervention with *CBITS*, the distress, anxiety, and depression suffered by children can be lifted and healed. The *CBITS* manual will also guide your work with parents and teachers with very positive results. One middle school teacher from Los Angeles said, "We thought we knew these kids pretty well but were surprised to find out the types of things they were carrying around with them. . . . Students benefited by having the time and opportunity to talk to a trained professional and identify problems we would normally not detect."

The effectiveness of *CBITS* can be discussed at length in the context of rigorous research design and evaluation. But, for me, the children's words are the most compelling evidence for the effectiveness of this intervention. The stories of the following three children (in their own words and in the words of their parents) show how they were positively impacted by CBITS.*

Jaime's Story

"Jaime," a seventh-grade student in a large middle school, was always worried about violence on his way to and from school. "I was walking home with a friend of mine and some other boys started following us and telling us stuff. They started threatening us and telling us they were going to hit us. They hit my friend. . . . I thought they were going to hit me too. . . . I realized that it's dangerous to walk home. . . ."

After ten sessions of the *CBITS* intervention, Jamie felt much more at ease. "I liked having the group here at school because it was easier for me to come. I wouldn't change anything because the group was fine how it was. . . . It helped me confront difficult things or times in my life. . . . Before the group, I hardly talked in class, but now I participate more."

Jaime's mother also saw positive changes in her son and in her family. "I notice that he's a bit different after the group. . . . He has more confidence in himself and he talks to us more about what he does at school and with his friends. As a family, we are more united, like a family should be. We talk more; we feel more comfortable with each other."

Will's Story

Violence in the community may sometimes mirror violence in the home. "Will," a ninth-grade student, had an encounter in a store with a man who was mentally ill. "He told me he wanted to kill me. . . . I ran to look for my mom. He was following me. I found a security guard and told him what was happening. Then I found my mother and told her. I was really scared. I didn't want to leave the house for a long time. I felt that crazy man knew where I lived."

All names have been changed to protect the privacy of the individuals.

Will's father believes both he and Will changed after using *CBITS*. "I feel Will has improved in school because he is now able to ask for help and also participates more. In terms of how it helped my family, well, I know that I used to be more aggressive with him. But now we are able to engage in conversations and have a good dialogue. I feel I can talk to him easier without losing my temper. The program was helpful to me as a parent. I can now talk with my son, and he can begin to feel that I, as his father, worry about him a lot."

George's Story

Sometimes, community violence involves the threat of weapons. Witnessing a violent criminal act terrorized "George," an elementary school student. "I was walking home from school with my cousin when I heard somebody screaming. We turned to see who it was and I saw a man being hit by four men. The men were wearing ski masks. We started to run. At that moment I heard gunshots. I was very afraid. When I was running I thought the men were following us. I thought that if they saw us they could look for us at school and hurt us. After that I was afraid to go to school. Everyday I tried a different path to go to and from school. I had nightmares."

The ten sessions of *CBITS* changed George's life at school for the better. "The group helped me because I don't have nightmares about that anymore. I liked the exercises. I like that I learned how to relax. I also liked being listened to. . . . I was able to do better at school because I had better concentration in class. I think this group is helpful for kids. . . . Kids can improve their grades, like I did, and get along with their teachers."

Children like George, Will, and Jaime are more and more prevalent in today's schools, making our work with children more important than ever. It is my hope that you will use *CBITS* to teach children new skills, help them experience success in the classroom, and ultimately, allow them to develop new hope and trust.

In July of 2003, the President's New Freedom Commission on Mental Health published its final report, *Achieving the Promise: Transforming Mental Health Care in America* (http://www.mentalhealthcommission.gov/reports/FinalReport/toc.html). It made several recommendations, including how to bring science to services, how to build the knowledge base needed for the treatment of trauma, and how to expand and enhance school-based mental health programs. It's aim was to change the mental health service delivery system in the United States so that adults and children with mental disorders can live, work, learn, and participate fully in their schools and communities.

CBITS brings these ideas together by providing an intervention that builds on the resilience of children to face life's challenges. It actively facilitates recovery and depends upon your skills and experience to bring it to life. I recommend this book for the mental health professionals who work in over 100,000 schools across the country. I know that you will find the *CBITS* manual helpful. This is a "must read" for the school counselor, school psychologist, or school social worker who is sincere in his or her commitment to bring science to practice.

Once again, I thank you for your commitment to providing quality services to children in schools. You have my admiration for your work and my appreciation for all you do to heal the hurt of psychological trauma.

Marleen Wong

Director
Crisis Counseling and Intervention Services
Los Angeles Unified School District

Director
School Crisis and Intervention Unit
National Center for Child Traumatic Stress
UCLA and Duke University

INTRODUCTION

In the last two decades, there has been an increasing awareness of the extent to which children are exposed to traumatic experiences (Pynoos et al., 1996). Between 20% and 50% of American children are victims of violence within their families, at school, or in their communities (Finkelhor & Dziuba-Leatherman, 1994). Increasing rates of community violence (Fitzpatrick & Boldizar, 1993; Richters & Martinez, 1993) have led public health officials to identify violence as one of the most significant public health issues facing America (Centers for Disease Control, 1990; Koop & Lundberg, 1992; Public Health Service, 1990). Studies have documented the broad range of negative sequelae of trauma exposure for children and adolescents, including problems such as post-traumatic stress disorder (PTSD) (Fitzpatrick & Boldizar, 1993; Jaycox et al., 2002; Martinez & Richters, 1993; Saigh & Bremner, 1999; Singer et al., 1995; Stein et al., 2001); other anxiety problems (Finkelhor, 1995; Osofsky et al., 1993; Singer et al., 1995); depressive symptoms (Jaycox et al., 2002; Kliewer et al., 1998; Martinez & Richters, 1993; Overstreet, 2000); dissociation (Putnam, 1997); impairment in school functioning (Garbarino et al., 1992; Hurt et al., 2001; Saigh et al., 1997; Schwab-Stone et al., 1995); decreased IQ and reading ability (Delaney-Black et al., 2002); lower grade-point average and more days of school absence (Hurt et al., 2001); and decreased rates of high school graduation (Grogger, 1997). Finally, trauma exposure is related to behavioral problems, particularly aggressive and delinquent behavior (Bell & Jenkins, 1991; Farrell & Bruce, 1997; Fitzpatrick & Boldizar, 1993; Garbarino et al., 1992; Jenkins & Bell, 1994; Martinez & Richters, 1993).

This manual is intended for use with groups of school children (ages 11–15) who have experienced significant traumatic experiences and are suffering from related emotional or behavioral problems, in particular, post-traumatic stress disorder or depression. Examples of traumatic life events include experiencing or witnessing severe violence, being in a natural or man-made disaster, experiencing a severe car accident or house fire, or being physically injured.

The *CBITS* manual is written for social workers, psychologists, psychiatrists, or school counselors with mental health intervention experience. Specialized training in cognitive-behavioral therapy and with trauma survivors is recommended. Because the program addresses sensitive issues and uses specific techniques, we do not recommend use by teachers or school staff who lack clinical training. Training in the use of these particular manuals is strongly encouraged. For more information, contact the author, Lisa Jaycox (jaycox@rand.org).

The program uses a skills-building, early intervention approach, and is therefore most appropriate for students with moderate levels of symptoms. The manual is especially focused on the reduction of symptoms of post-traumatic stress disorder (PTSD). Since depression and diffuse anxiety often accompany symptoms of PTSD, many of the techniques in this manual are targeted toward depressive and general anxiety symptoms as well. Though focused primarily on students with moderate distress, youths with a diagnosed mental disorder such as PTSD would also be expected to benefit from this program. However, such students will most likely require concurrent individual therapy as well as a referral for continued treatment after the *CBITS* group ends.

This book has three parts that are intended to be used concurrently:

- ❏ The child group and individual program (ten group sessions and one to three individual sessions).
- ❏ The parent education program (two sessions).
- ❏ The teacher education program (one session).

For each, there are detailed instructions for presenting material to the groups, as well as informational handouts and worksheets.

We recommend that this program be implemented in the following manner:

1. Select the school and population of students to be included.

2. Determine the permissions that will be required for students to participate in the program. Active parental consent is usually required.

3. Identify the teachers that will be impacted by the program, and whose students will be included, and ask them to participate in the teacher education program.

4. After obtaining the appropriate permissions, identify youth for inclusion in the program through a student screening procedure.

5. Meet with selected students to confirm that the program is appropriate for them; meet with parents and conduct assessments.

6. Assess the children to be included and begin the child program.

7. Implement the parent education program as the child groups begin, within the first half of the child group

program. These often need to be held in the late afternoon or evening to accommodate parent schedules.

8. After the child program ends, conduct another assessment to determine improvements in symptoms, and make referrals for continued care as warranted.

Selection of Participants

CBITS is intended for youth, ages 11–15 who have experienced a significant trauma and who have significant symptoms of post-traumatic stress disorder or depression. We recommend using a screening instrument in the general school population in order to identify children in need of this program. There are several standard scales that could be used to identify children (see Cohen, 1998). First, you will need to screen for exposure to a significant traumatic event. In our work, we focused on community violence and used a scale that included exposure to specific acts of violence (Singer et al., 1995; Singer et al., 1998). Second, you will need two measures of symptoms (post-traumatic stress disorder and depression) that provide validated cut-offs for scores that indicate a significant or clinical level of severity. We used the Child PTSD Symptom Scale (Foa et al., 2001) and the Children's Depression Scale (Kovacs, 1981). Since children's responses on self-report measures are not always valid, it is important to follow up the screening process with a personal interview in which their responses are reviewed and confirmed by a clinician. If the child does not appear to be symptomatic during this interview, it is important to follow up with parents or teachers to validate the interview and make a joint decision about inclusion or exclusion from the *CBITS* group.

In inner city schools, it is expected that many students (upwards of 20%) would benefit from this kind of intervention. In other areas, the proportion of students who would benefit may be less. If the entire school is affected by a disaster or violence, it is possible that many more than 20% would benefit from this kind of intervention. In these cases, school counselors should wait three to six months after the trauma before identifying those in need.

Evaluation of *CBITS*

CBITS was developed in collaboration with the Los Angeles Unified School District. We pilot-tested the program in one of their clinics for clinic-referred children and then conducted two research studies. We updated the manual several times during this period, based on feedback from social workers, students, and parents. Several publications describe the nature of our partnership and the development of the intervention model as well as the results of our screening of children who had recently immigrated (Jaycox et al., 2002; Stein et al., 2002).

In the first study, we screened 879 children who were Spanish-speaking, recent immigrants between the ages of 8 and 15. We found that 31% had trauma experiences and current symptoms, making them eligible to be in the program. Of this 31%, 83% consented to participate in the program and research study, and had parent permission to do so. Seventy-two percent of those with consent completed the program and an assessment following it, for a total of 198 participants. Students in the intervention group (n = 152) had significantly greater improvement in PTSD and depressive symptoms compared to those on the waitlist (n = 46) at a three-month follow-up, adjusting for relevant covariates (Kataoka et al., 2003).

In the second study, we screened 769 students in the general school population between the ages of 10 and 12. Using slightly more stringent criteria for inclusion than in the first study, we determined that 159 (21%) were appropriate for inclusion in the program. Of these, 126 agreed to participate and remained in the area, and were therefore randomized into the study. Results show that those in the intervention group had reduced self-reported symptoms of PTSD and depression at post-test, as well as reduced parent-reported behavioral and emotional problems (Stein et al., 2003).

BACKGROUND ON *CBITS* FOR GROUP LEADERS

What is cognitive-behavioral therapy (CBT)? Cognitive-behavioral therapy is a structured, symptom-focused therapy that includes a wide variety of skill-building techniques. All are based on the premise that thoughts and behaviors can cause negative emotions and patterns of interactions with others. Making maladaptive thoughts and behaviors more functional is the goal of CBT. Thus, techniques are geared toward changing maladaptive thoughts (challenging negative thinking, stopping automatic negative thoughts, distracting from negative patterns of thinking) and behaviors (improving social skills, increasing pleasant activities, decreasing avoidance of difficult situations or thoughts). Several structural characteristics of the therapy tend to differentiate it from other types of therapy. These include:

- ❑ **Structured sessions.** An agenda is set for each session that includes activities review, new skills or practice with skills, and activities assignment.

- ❑ **Collaboration between patient and therapist.** The therapist acts as a "coach" to help the patient develop new skills and to find ways to practice them effectively.

- ❑ **Emphasis on practice of new techniques during sessions and between sessions.** Activities are assigned between sessions and are important for consolidating skills learned in-group.

- ❑ **Short-term interventions.** The goal is to enable the patient to continue practice on his or her own after the intervention ends.

What symptoms are addressed by *CBITS*? This set of manuals is intended for use with groups of children who have experienced significant traumatic experiences and are suffering from symptoms of post-traumatic stress disorder. Since depression and diffuse anxiety often accompany symptoms of PTSD, many of the techniques are targeted toward depressive and general anxiety symptoms as well. This intervention is designed especially for youths with moderate levels of symptoms, with or without diagnosable PTSD. Youths with a diagnosis of severe PTSD are expected to benefit from the *CBITS* as well but may need additional individual treatment to augment the procedures and lengthen the duration of stress- or trauma-focused work.

What is PTSD? Post-traumatic stress disorder (PTSD) is an anxiety disorder that develops following exposure to an extreme stressor. It includes the following types of symptoms: re-experiencing of the traumatic event (nightmares, recurrent thoughts), avoidance of trauma reminders (avoidance of thoughts, feelings, and situations that remind one of the trauma; emotional numbing), and arousal (irritability, difficulty sleeping and concentrating, hypervigilance). PTSD symptoms can create severe problems with everyday functioning and often co-occur with symptoms of depression, substance abuse, and behavioral problems.

What age groups benefit from CBITS? This *CBITS* program is designed for youth, ages 11–15. It is desirable to group children close in age together if possible (e.g., younger children, ages 11–13; older children, ages 13–15).

What skills are taught by *CBITS*? An outline of the new concepts taught in each session is listed in **Table 1**. A rationale for each major technique follows **Table 1**.

Table 1: Session Outline

Child Group and Individual Program	
Group Session 1:	**Introduction of group members, confidentiality, and group procedures.** • Explanation of treatment using stories. • Discussion of reasons for participation (kinds of stress or trauma).
Group Session 2:	**Education about common reactions to stress or trauma.** • Relaxation training to combat anxiety.
Individual Sessions:	**Between Session 2 and Session 6.** • Imaginal exposure to traumatic event.
Group Session 3:	**Thoughts and feelings (Introduction to cognitive therapy).** • Fear Thermometer. • Linkage between thoughts and feelings. • Combating negative thoughts.
Group Session 4:	**Combating negative thoughts.**
Group Session 5:	**Avoidance and coping (Introduction to real life exposure).** • Construction of fear hierarchy. • Alternative coping strategies.
Group Session 6:	**Exposure to stress or trauma memory through imagination/drawing/ writing.**
Group Session 7:	**Exposure to stress or trauma memory through imagination/drawing/ writing.**
Group Session 8:	**Introduction to social problem-solving.**
Group Session 9:	**Practice with social problem-solving and Hot Seat.**
Group Session 10:	**Relapse prevention and graduation ceremony.**
Parent Education Program	
Session 1:	**Education about reactions to trauma, how we explain fear, relaxation.**
Session 2:	**How we teach children to change their thoughts and actions.**
Teacher Education Program	
Education about reactions to trauma, elements of the *CBITS* program, tips for teaching youth who have been traumatized.	

Rationale for Components of the Intervention

CBITS teaches six techniques:

- ❑ Education
- ❑ Relaxation training
- ❑ Cognitive therapy
- ❑ Real life exposure
- ❑ Stress or trauma exposure
- ❑ Social problem-solving.

Education: The sessions begin with a presentation of the model that will be used throughout the intervention. The model stresses feelings, thoughts, and actions, all of which have an impact on each other. This model is derived from one used to treat adult depression (Lewinsohn et al., 1986). Since many symptoms emerge following stress or trauma, the traumatized individual can often feel out of control and demoralized about being "weak" or "unable to cope." Psychoeducation, therefore, can be very useful in destigmatizing the symptoms of anxiety, anger, and grief that follow stress or trauma. In addition, it is a useful way to introduce the concept of PTSD as a disorder that can be treated, rather than an out-of-control set of symptoms that will last forever. In *CBITS*, children are educated in a group format, a handout is sent home to parents, and a call to parents at the beginning of treatment is used to answer questions and reinforce the ideas in the handout. This process follows that used in treatment of adults with PTSD (Foa et al., 1994a; Foa et al., 1994b). Parent education occurs via a handout sent before Group Session 2, and child education occurs in Group Sessions 1 and 2.

Relaxation Training: Relaxation training is used to combat anxiety. Controlled breathing and progressive muscle relaxation are taught in session and practiced periodically during the treatment. Such training has the benefit of reducing anxiety and giving the trainee a sense of control over anxiety symptoms. In addition, the same techniques can be used to manage anger. These techniques are taught in Group Session 2.

Cognitive Therapy: Studies of adults and preliminary work with children have provided evidence for the idea that stress or trauma changes some of the primary assumptions made about the self and the world. Specifically, traumatized individuals tend to believe that the world is more dangerous and that they themselves are less competent following a stress or trauma (see Foa & Jaycox, 1999, for a review). Cognitive theory holds that such maladaptive thoughts cause and maintain emotional disturbances, and cognitive therapy aims to correct erroneous assumptions so that more flexibility and accuracy in thinking is accomplished. These two themes (world dangerousness and personal incompetence) will be explored via cognitive therapy, and children are taught to recognize these sorts of maladaptive thoughts and to combat them by replacing them with more realistic appraisals of danger and competence. The sessions follow the structure of a program for depressed children (Gillham et al., 1991; Gillham et al., 1995; Jaycox et al., 1994) and modified for use with adolescents (Asarnow et al., 1999a and 1999b). These techniques are introduced in Group Session 3 and practiced in the remaining sessions through activities between sessions and games during the sessions.

Real Life Exposure: Real life exposure, one of the cornerstones of behavioral treatment for anxiety disorders, is a method in which patients are gradually exposed to feared situations in order to reduce anxiety. This method capitalizes on habituation, the process by which anxiety decreases when a feared situation is confronted without actual danger. In *CBITS*, children are helped to construct a list of situations that they fear as a result of their traumatic experiences and are encouraged to confront such situations in a controlled fashion with the help of their parents. Planning for this exercise occurs in Group Session 5, and review and practice takes place in the subsequent group sessions. Special emphasis is put on setting goals for these exercises that do not expose children to any real danger. For instance, an assignment might be to look at a picture of an event similar to the one that caused the trauma or to go to the scene of the traumatic event, if it isn't dangerous. If no exercises can be identified that provide safety and parental supervision, participants are encouraged to practice alternative coping strategies. These include distraction, thought stopping, positive imagery, and relaxation, and follow Stress Inoculation Training models for adults (Kilpatrick et al., 1982) and of coping skills programs for children (e.g., Gillham et al., 1991).

Stress or Trauma Exposure: Imaginal or creative exposure to stress or trauma memories is a hallmark of cognitive-behavioral therapy for PTSD. Just as real life exposure decreases anxiety around stress or trauma reminders, imaginal exposure decreases the intense anxiety and discomfort that accompany memories of the event (Foa & Jaycox, 1999). In the *CBITS* program, following the model of March and colleagues (March et al., 1998), the first exposure to the stress or trauma memory, which can be upsetting, occurs in the privacy of the individual therapy session. Subsequent exposures to the memory take place in-group, through drawings of the event and descriptions of the drawings to the group. All exposures are paced according to the needs of the individual children so that they do not feel overwhelmed or overly upset when they work on this exercise. Feelings of grief are also emphasized during this segment of the program so that children are able to express and cope with grief reactions related to the stress or trauma. In addition, during the individual sessions, children are asked what kind of support they would like from peers in the group and are coached on ways to support others during the group exposure process.

Social Problem-Solving: Standard social problem-solving techniques are taught to combat the anger and impulsivity that can follow a traumatic event and to improve management of current real life problems. Social problem-solving is introduced using an approach to "healthy management of reality" used with adults (Muñoz & Miranda, 1986) and adapted for adolescents (Asarnow et al., 1999a and 1999b). Following the format of a child depression program (Gillham et al., 1991), these techniques help children slow down their reactions in interpersonal situations, evaluate their options and goals for the encounters, and choose the behaviors that they think will work best. Examples and role-playing are used to reinforce these techniques in the group format. These techniques are introduced in Session 8 and practiced in the remaining sessions.

Program Format

Activities Assignments and Review: Activities are an essential element to the *CBITS* intervention, as they consolidate skills and allow group members to apply these skills to their real life problems. It is very important to leave sufficient time in each session to review activities assigned in the previous session and to explain and assign activities for the subsequent session. In reviewing activities, counselors should attempt to identify problem areas with children and to make sure that this problem area gets addressed during the group or in a subsequent activities assignment. During activities assignments, counselors should review the individual goals of each group member to clear up any confusion and to make sure that group members are setting realistic, achievable goals. It can be very gratifying for group members to have teachers collect their activities, review them, and write some encouraging and positive comments.

Practice of Intervention Techniques: Ideally, once a technique is taught in the group, group members will practice it in and between sessions for the rest of the program. However, as the number of techniques builds, it becomes unmanageable to assign all techniques as activities. Instead, group members should be encouraged to use all the techniques available when activities are assigned and reviewed and practice techniques that were taught earlier whenever there is time or opportunity. For instance, Hot Seat exercises can be done any time that there is extra time in the group session.

Individual Treatment Planning: Although *CBITS* is presented in a group format, it is still important to conceptualize each individual "case" and to gear the program toward the individuals in the group. Group members' needs should always be the priority over following the manual in strict terms. In addition, choosing group members to participate at each point in the program should be guided by group members' needs. See the list of problem areas and program components in **Table 2**:

Table 2: How to match needs to techniques.

Problem Area	Program Component
Severe general anxiety	Relaxation, alternative coping strategies
Nightmares, flashbacks, intrusive thinking	Exposure to the stress or traumatic event
Severe situational anxiety	Real life exposure, cognitive therapy
Avoidance of stress or trauma reminders	Real life exposure
Guilt	Cognitive therapy
Shame	Exposure to the stress or traumatic event
Grief/sadness/loss	Exposure to stress or traumatic event (grief focus)
Poor self-concept	Cognitive therapy, real life exposure
Problems with peers or family	Social problem-solving
Impulsivity	Social problem-solving

The *Case Formulation Worksheet* (Appendix A) facilitates the conceptualization of needs for each participant. We recommend that group leaders complete this worksheet for each participant prior to the initial group sessions. Review and modify the individual worksheets during supervision and periodically throughout treatment.

Group Format and Management: Child group sessions are formatted to last approximately one hour. The usual format is to convene groups of identified children during the school day, preferably during a nonacademic period. Groups can also be held after school if obstacles such as transportation concerns can be addressed. Groups are usually held once per week. In some groups, it is helpful to write an outline on the chalkboard at the beginning of the session. It may also be useful to develop a point system to increase activities participation and then to reward the

group members who complete the most activities or to provide incentives for activities participation throughout the program. Any such group management techniques can be implemented to augment group participation and compliance.

Materials Needed: Notebooks containing the program handouts should be created for the participants and extra copies made in case children lose or misplace their notebooks. For each session, have a chalkboard or large writing pad and extra copies of the activity worksheets for the session. A bag of M&M's® candies or something similar is required for Session 1. Depending on the time of the intervention, it could be important to provide a snack or drinks for the participants.

Individual Sessions: Because of the sensitive nature of talking about traumatic events, *CBITS* includes a required individual session with each child. Individual sessions are to be held sometime between Group Sessions 2 and 6. These individual sessions are arranged separately with each child and last about one hour or less. The purpose of the individual session is threefold: (1) to gather information about the trauma that will be useful in planning the intervention; (2) to conduct exposure to the trauma memory; and (3) to help the child plan the exposures that he or she will do in Group Sessions 6 and 7. At the end of the first individual session, decide if the session has been sufficient to fulfill these three purposes. If not, schedule an additional one or two individual sessions.

Parent Participation: Parents are not involved in the group itself but should be engaged as much as possible through telephone contact and parent education sessions. The first phone call to parents should occur at the beginning of therapy, preferably before the group sessions begin, but at a minimum before Group Session 2. During this call, describe common reactions to stress or trauma, explain the therapy and its procedures, and enlist parental help with activity assignments and session attendance. Subsequent phone calls can be made as needed. They are often helpful in preparation for the real life exposure activities in Group Session 5 and can also be a review of progress and suggest additional treatment if necessary.

Special Issues in Working with Stress or Trauma Survivors

Working with stress or trauma survivors requires sensitivity and patience. There are several points that are important to keep in mind:

❑ Children who have been exposed to violence and who are symptomatic may be guarded and slow to trust. Careful explanation of group procedures and rationales for all the components of the program can help to build trust and gain compliance. Make sure that all group members understand the concept of confidentiality, and try to build a cohesive group that feels safe to all group members.

❑ Such children may overreact to real or perceived injustices, so group leaders need to be consistent and predictable.

❑ There are a wide variety of symptoms that can be expressed, and some of them can be hard to deal with as a group leader. Try to view all the symptoms as adaptive, creative ways that the children have learned in order to cope with devastating events.

❑ Children often tend to "reenact" the stress or trauma, and can sometimes try to provoke adults into being abusive. Don't fall into this trap. Check your own anger and frustration often, and make sure that you do not feed into the cycle of abuse that the children are accustomed to in any way.

❑ Children who have been traumatized get scared easily. Be conservative in the use of physical contact, and always ask permission before unexpectedly touching a group member (unless it is a matter of safety).

Working with Children Who Have Been Multiply Traumatized: This book takes an approach to children in relation to a single traumatic event. However, it is more typical for children to have experienced several traumatic events of different types at various points in their lives. Therefore, some treatment planning is necessary. Consider with the children which event is most troublesome at present, and concentrate on that event first. As symptoms related to that event begin to subside, turn to less troublesome events. You may find it possible to work on several events with some children and on just one event with others. Specific instructions for choosing which traumatic event to focus on are included in the relevant sections.

Child Group and Individual Program

INTRODUCTIONS

I. Introduction to the Group

Meeting Schedule

Review the meeting schedule, and pass out written schedules for the children to take home. Talk about the importance of being on time to show respect for other group members and to review their between-session practice. Make sure that group members understand that each session builds on the one before it and that it is important to make it to all of the sessions.

Confidentiality

Review the concept of confidentiality, and elicit from group members reasons why they might want the group to be private. Request that group members keep everything that is talked about in the group private, but allow group members to talk about their own participation with anyone that they want. Review a few examples to make sure that everyone understands:

"Let's say that there is a boy named Joe in this group. If Joe were to tell everyone in the group that he has been fighting a lot with his brother, would it be okay to tell a classmate at school that he said that? Why not?"

"Would it be okay to tell a classmate at school who the others in the group are and why they are in the group? Why not?"

A G E N D A	**I. Introduction to the Group**
	  A. Meeting Schedule
	  B. Confidentiality
	  C. Introduction Game
	II. Explanation of *CBITS*
	III. Why We Are Here: Our Stories
	IV. Activities Assignment

OBJECTIVES
1. Build group cohesion.
2. Reduce anxiety about participating in the group.

SPECIAL SUPPLIES
1. M&M's candies
2. Confidentiality statement (optional)
3. Index cards
4. Copies of the "Goals" worksheet

"If I feel upset after the group, would it be okay for me to tell my mother what it was that made me upset? Why?"

It may be a good idea to have group members sign a statement saying that they will keep what others say in the group private, to ensure that they are taking this issue seriously.

Introduction Game: The M&M's Game[1]

Pass around a bag of M&M's, and tell each child to take a small handful but not to eat them. Tell them that you are going to ask them some questions about themselves and that everyone who has a certain color M&M in their hand has to answer the question in front of the group before they can eat it. For example:

---

[1] This game was modified from one originally used in Gillham, J., Jaycox, L. H., Reivich, K. J., Seligman, M. E. P., & Silver, T. (1991). *Manual for Leaders of the Coping Skills Program for Children.* Unpublished manual. Copyright Foresight, Inc.

"This is for anyone who has a blue M&M: What do you do for fun after school?"

Model an appropriate answer yourself first, and play along so that they can get to know you as well. If the children have more than one blue M&M, they must tell you one thing for each one. Other possible questions include:

"What kind of job would you like to have after you finish school?"

"What sports or physical activities are you good at?"

"When do you have fun during the school day?"

Write questions on index cards before the session for easy use during the game. You can then give one of the children an index card and ask him or her to read the question aloud to increase group participation.

The goal of this game is to build group rapport and to get the group members used to sharing personal information. Try to use questions that will be relevant and interesting to the group (depending on age, gender, maturity), but avoid questions that will lead to too much self-disclosure at this early stage in the group.

II. Explanation of *CBITS*

Give an overview of the idea that thoughts and behaviors influence the way we feel. Draw a triangle on the board. Write the phrase "Stress or Trauma" to one side, with an arrow pointing at the triangle (see **Figure 1**). Then say:

"What do I mean by stress or trauma? Can you give some examples of things that might happen that would be stressful?"

Elicit ideas about stressful events, and list under the "Stress or Trauma" heading. Then ask:

"When something stressful happens [use one of their examples], how does that change what we think? What we do? What we feel?"

Make the point that stress or trauma causes all three aspects to change and that each then impacts the others, making feelings worsen. A possible example:

"You get into a car accident. That's the stress or trauma. Afterwards, you feel shaky, nervous, upset. You think that driving is really dangerous, and you don't want to go in the car again. When your mother asks if you want to go shopping with her, you say no and stay home because you don't want to be in the car."

Using a made-up name in this example can be useful. As the group progresses, you can refer back to the named person when explaining what you are working on. (For instance, Session 3 could be introduced this way: "Remember George, who was in that car accident? Remember how George thought about what happened to him? Well, today, we're going to work on changing that kind of thinking.")

Explain how *CBITS* is going to help the children cope with upsetting things:

"You are all here because you had something really stressful happen to you. In this program, we are going to work on all three corners of the triangle. We are going to:

- *Learn some exercises that will make you FEEL better, and less nervous or upset.*

- *Learn some ways to THINK about things that will help you feel better.*

- *Learn some ways to DO things so that you are able to do everything you want to be able to do and not feel upset when you do it."*

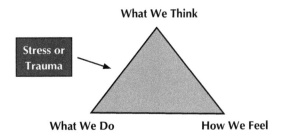

Figure 1

III. Why We Are Here: Our Stories

Use this section to introduce the reasons for each group member's participation. You will want to limit self-disclosure at this point. The goal is for group members to talk very briefly about why they are in the group but not leave the group feeling upset. Begin with this explanation:

"Let's spend a few minutes talking about the biggest stress or trauma each of you went through, the one that brought you into the group. It can sometimes be upsetting to talk about stresses or traumas, and we don't want you to feel upset today. So please just share a very little bit of what happened to you so that the others in the group have an idea, but not so much that you start to feel upset about it. If anyone wants help from me in telling the group what happened, let me know, and I'll say it for you. If more than one thing happened to you, tell us about the different things and which one bothers you the most now."

Spend a minute or two allowing each group member to tell the others about the event or events that brought him or her into the group. For those with more than one event, ask them to tell the group which one bothers them the most at present. If a child says that all are equal, ask which one was the most difficult at the time that it happened. Take notes about the relevant trauma for each child so that you can refer to them later in the program.

At the end, summarize the kinds of experiences for the group, emphasizing commonalities. For instance:

"This shows us that everyone has had something really stressful happen. Every one of you had a different thing happen, but it seems like a few/several/all of you went through something that was very scary/where someone might have been hurt/that was really startling or shocking/where you didn't have any control over what happened. We're going to work on making these stresses or traumas easier for you to deal with."

IV. Activities Assignment

Describe the activities assignment of setting goals for therapy. Distribute copies of the following "Goals" worksheet and have the children begin to work on it if there is time. Tell them to share their worksheets with their parents and ask their parent to complete the bottom section. Have them bring the worksheets to the next group session.

GOALS

Name: _____

Section: _____

BY THE END OF THIS GROUP,

I want to feel LESS:

❑ Nervous   ❑ Scared   ❑ Angry   ❑ Upset   ❑ Sad

I want to feel MORE:

❑ Happy   ❑ Calm   ❑ Excited   ❑ Relaxed

I want to change the way I do things and think about things so that I can:

❑ Calm myself down when I feel upset.

❑ Think about things that happened without feeling upset.

❑ Talk about things that happened without feeling upset.

❑ Stop avoiding things that make me nervous.

❑ Do more of the things that I used to do.

❑ Think more about things before I do them.

❑ Make better decisions.

❑ Have fewer problems with my family.

❑ Have fewer problems with my friends.

I also want to change:

_____

_____

_____

_____

– –

Parent's Section

What would you like to see changed in your child by the end of the group?

_____

_____

_____

EDUCATION AND RELAXATION

I. Activities Review

Review each group member's "Goals" Worksheet by asking for volunteers to share their goals. Reassure group members that goals are attainable and remind them about the ways in which you will help them with each goal. At the same time, point out which goals are unrealistic, and help group members understand how they can begin work on some goals in group session and then continue to work on them on their own afterwards. The overall tone of this part of the session should convey a realistic, hopeful attitude.

If some group members did not have their parents complete the worksheet or did not want to share it with their parents, normalize that for them ("Yes, parents can be busy, and it can be hard to get this done," or "Yes, sometimes these things feel too private to share with others"). This will help ensure that they are not embarrassed in front of the group.

II. Education About Common Reactions to Trauma

Take some time to convey information about general types of problems that children experience when they have been exposed to traumatic life events. The goal is to normalize symptoms. In groups of older children, this can be presented in a group discussion format, by writing the problem on the board and then having group members describe what that problem is like for them. In a younger group, write the problems on slips of paper or index cards and put them in a hat.

AGENDA

I. Activities Review
II. Education About Common Reactions to Trauma
III. Relaxation Training to Combat Anxiety
IV. Activities Assignment

OBJECTIVES
1. Reduce stigma about trauma-related symptoms.
2. Build peer support.
3. Increase parent-child communication and support.
4. Build skills: Relaxation.

SPECIAL SUPPLIES
1. Index cards and hat (optional)
2. Highlighters (optional)
3. Copies of the "Handout for Parents"
4. Copies of the "Activities" worksheet

Have each group member pick a problem and describe what it's like for him or her. Have other group members add their experiences as well, and then move on to another group member.

Alternative approach: Pass out colored highlighter pens and ask group members to turn to the list of common reactions in the "Activities" worksheet (at the end of the Group Session 2 section). Ask them to highlight the parts that apply to themselves.

If group members add additional problems to the list, adopt an accepting attitude and try to make the connections to the traumatic events. If there are no apparent connections, gently remind the group members that there are all sorts of problems, but only those that stem from stress and trauma will be discussed in the group. Since the goal is to normalize symptoms, an inclusive discussion that includes all sorts of problems is best. Adding comments to the group members' experiences (examples follow) will help to normalize the symptoms and provide hope that they can be reduced in the group.

Common Reactions to Stress or Trauma

When stress or trauma occurs, people cope in different ways. Describe to the group the most common reactions to trauma.

Having nightmares or trouble sleeping. When something really scary or upsetting happens, it takes awhile to figure out exactly what happened and what it means. After severe stress or trauma, people tend to keep thinking about what happened in order to "digest" it, just like your stomach has to work to digest a big meal. This can take a long time. Nightmares are one way of digesting what happened to you.

Thinking about it all the time. This is another way to digest what happened. Just like having nightmares, thinking about the trauma all the time is a problem because it makes you feel upset. It can be unpleasant.

Wanting to NOT think or talk about it. This is natural, since it is upsetting to think about a past stress or trauma, and it can make you feel all sorts of emotions. Avoiding it makes things easier, but only for a little while. It's important to digest what happened sooner or later. So, while avoiding it sometimes makes sense, you have to set aside some time to digest it also. This group can be the time and place you set aside to digest what happened to you.

Avoiding places, people, or things that make you think about it. Just like not wanting to talk about or think about the trauma, avoiding situations that remind you of what happened can help you feel better right then. The problem with this, though, is that it keeps you from doing normal things that are an impor-

tant part of your life. The goal of this group is to get you back to the point where you are able to do whatever you want to do, without worrying about whether it will remind you of what happened.

Feeling scared for no reason. Sometimes this happens because you remember what happened to you, or you are thinking about what happened. Other times it happens because your body is so tense all the time that you just start feeling scared. Either way, we can work on helping you feel calmer when it happens.

Feeling "crazy" or out of control. If all of these things are problems for you, you can start to feel really out of control or even crazy. Don't worry, though; these problems don't mean that you are going crazy. They are all normal reactions to stress or trauma, and there are ways to help you feel better.

Not being able to remember parts of what happened. This happens to a lot of people. The stressful event can be so awful that your memory doesn't work the way it usually does. Sometimes it gets easier to remember later on, and sometimes it gets harder. This can be frustrating, but it is really normal.

Having trouble concentrating at school or at home. With all the nervousness you are feeling and all the time you are spending thinking about what happened, it can be hard to concentrate on school work or even on what your friends or family say to you.

Being on guard to protect yourself; feeling like something bad is about to happen. After something bad happens to you, it makes sense to be prepared for another bad thing to happen. The problem with this is that you can spend so much time waiting for the next bad thing to happen that you don't have time or energy for other things in your life. Also, it is scary to think something bad is going to happen.

Jumping when there is a loud noise. This is one way that your body says it is prepared for action, in case something else happens. As you begin to feel calmer, this will go away.

Feeling anger. Some people feel angry about the stress or trauma that happened, or about the things that happened afterward. Other people just feel angry all the time, at everything and everybody. Both of these are normal and will get better as you begin to digest what happened to you.

Feeling shame. Sometimes people are ashamed about what happened to them or how they acted. Even though it's hard to believe, this gets better the more that you talk about what happened. If you keep it a secret, it's hard for the shame to go away.

Feeling guilt. People can feel guilty about what happened or about something they did or did not do. Sometimes you blame yourself for things that you couldn't control. You may also feel guilty for upsetting your parents. Guilty feelings can make it hard to talk about what happened.

Feeling sadness/grief/loss. Sometimes stress events or traumas include losing someone close to you or losing something that is important to you. This makes you feel sad and down. We'll help you talk about these feelings in the group.

Feeling bad about yourself. Sometimes, all this stress can make you feel really bad about yourself, like you're a bad person or that no one likes you. This makes it harder to be friendly and to have fun with others.

Having physical health problems and complaints. Stress has an effect on your body as well. People sometimes get sick more often or notice pain and discomfort more often when they have been under stress.

At the end of the discussion, summarize for the group that people feel many different things but that all are normal. Use the information gleaned during this discussion to guide the program for each individual group member, focusing practice of relevant techniques on the group members who need that technique the most.

III. Relaxation Training to Combat Anxiety

The goal of this part of the session is to train group members in progressive muscle relaxation. Present the following rationale:

"Stress makes our bodies tense, and feeling nervous or upset makes it even worse. But there are ways to relax your body that will make you feel calmer. Today, I'll teach you one way to do that."

Ask group members to lean back in their chairs (or lie on the floor if that is more comfortable), close their eyes, and follow your instructions. Giggling is common among children doing relaxation exercises. Warn them that they might find it funny at first, but that they should try to relax and concentrate on your voice. If group members have trouble staying focused, move over to them one by one and put your hand on their shoulder to help them focus. (If, however, the group member is jumpy, warn him or her that you will touch a shoulder before you do it.) Guide the children:

"I'd like you to start by thinking of someplace that makes you really comfortable, like your bed or the bathtub or the couch or the beach. Imagine that you are lying down there or sitting comfortably. Take a breath in [wait 3–4 seconds] and out [wait 3–4 seconds], in . . . and out . . . in . . . and out. Try to keep breathing this way as we continue. And keep thinking about your most comfortable spot.

"Now I'd like you to make a fist and squeeze it really tight. You can open your eyes and see how I'm doing it if you're not sure how. Hold it. Now relax it completely, and shake it out. Do it again; make a fist. Now relax it completely. Can you feel the difference between how it was when it was tight and now how it feels when it's relaxed? Let's do the same thing for the rest of your arms. Tighten up your whole arm, like you are making a muscle, and hold it. Now relax it completely. Do it again. Tighten, now relax. Now let's move to your shoulders. Bring your shoulders up to your ears and tighten them . . . hold it. Now relax. Do that again. Bring your shoulders way up near your ears . . . hold it . . . now relax it completely. Make sure your hands, arms, and shoulders are completely relaxed. Breathe in . . . and out . . . in . . . and out.

"Let's work on your face now. Scrunch up your face as tight as you can, close your eyes tight, scrunch up your mouth, and hold it. Now relax. Try that again. Tighten up your whole face, and hold it. Now relax it. Keep breathing like we did before . . . in . . . and out . . . in . . . and out.

Next comes your body. Arch your back as much as you can, and put your shoulders way back, like I am doing. Hold it. Now relax that. Next, lean forward onto your knees and curl your back the other way, and tighten up your stomach as much as you can. Hold it. Now relax it. Do that again . . . hold it, and relax it. Keep breathing . . . in . . . and out . . . in . . . and out.

"Let's work on your legs and feet. Straighten your legs up in the air in front of you and bring your toes as close to your face as you can. Tighten up your bottom also. Now hold it. Relax. Do that again . . . hold it, and now relax. Next, point your toes as far as you can away from your face, and again tighten up your leg muscles. Hold it. Now relax. Do that again . . . hold it, and relax. Breath in . . . and out . . . in . . . and out.

"Think about all the parts of your body, and relax any part that is tight now. Let all the tension go out of your body. Breathe in . . . and out . . . in . . . and out. Now begin to open your eyes, sit back up, and be a part of the group again."

IV. Activities Assignment

There are two activity assignments:

1. Give group members copies of the "Handout for Parents" about common reactions to stress or trauma, and ask them to talk with their parents about the problems bothering them.

2. Tell group members to practice the relaxation exercise three times, before going to bed.

Distribute copies of the "Activities" worksheet. Ask the children to fill them out and bring them to the next session.

Name: _____

COMMON REACTIONS TO STRESS OR TRAUMA

Show this to your parents. Tell them which things are bothering you.

There are many different ways that young people react to stressful life events. Below we've listed several kinds of reactions, all of which are very common. We've asked your child to show this list to you and to talk with you about which ones he or she has had problems with recently. You might also notice the way that you've reacted to stressful events in your own life. Feel free to call us if you have any questions about these problems or the way in which the group will address them.

Having nightmares or trouble sleeping. When something really scary or upsetting happens, it takes awhile to figure out exactly what happened and what it means. After severe stress or trauma, people tend to keep thinking about what happened in order to "digest" it, just like your stomach has to work to digest a big meal. Nightmares are one way of digesting what happened.

Thinking about it all the time. This is another way to digest what happened. Just like nightmares, thinking about the trauma all the time is a problem because it makes you feel upset. It can be unpleasant.

Wanting to NOT think or talk about it. This is natural, since it is upsetting to think about a past stress or trauma, and it can make you feel all sorts of emotions. Avoiding it makes things easier, but only for a little while. It's important to digest what happened sooner or later. So, while avoiding it sometimes makes sense, you have to set aside some time to digest it also.

Avoiding places, people, or things that make you think about it. Just like not wanting to talk about or think about the trauma, avoiding situations that remind you of what happened can

help you feel better right then. The problem with this, though, is that it keeps you from doing normal things that are an important part of your life.

Feeling scared for no reason. Sometimes this happens because you remember what happened to you, or you are thinking about what happened. Other times it happens because your body is so tense all the time that you just start feeling scared.

Feeling "crazy" or out of control. If all of these things are problems for you, you can start to feel really out of control or even crazy. Don't worry, though; these problems don't mean that you are going crazy. They are all common reactions to stress or trauma.

Not being able to remember parts of what happened. This happens to a lot of people. The stressful event can be so awful that your memory doesn't work the way it usually does. Sometimes it gets easier to remember it later on, and sometimes it gets harder. This can be frustrating, but it's really normal.

Having trouble concentrating at school or at home. With all the nervousness you are feeling and all the time you are spending thinking about what happened, it can be hard to concentrate on school work or even what your friends or family say to you.

Being on guard to protect yourself; feeling like something bad is about to happen. After something bad happens to you, it makes sense to be prepared for another bad thing to happen. The problem with this is that you can spend so much time waiting for the next bad thing to happen that you don't have time or energy for other things in your life. Also, it is scary to think something bad is going to happen all the time.

Jumping when there is a loud noise. This is another way to say that your body is prepared for action, in case something else happens.

Feeling anger. Sometimes people feel angry about the stress or trauma that happened, or the things that happened afterward. Other times, people just feel angry all the time, at everything and everybody.

Feeling shame. Sometimes people are ashamed about what happened to them, or how they acted. Even though it's hard to believe, this gets better the more that you talk about what hap-

pened. If you keep it a secret, it's hard for the shame to go away.

Feeling guilt. People can feel guilty about what happened or about something they did or did not do. Sometimes you blame yourself for things that you couldn't control. You may also feel guilty for upsetting other people. Guilty feelings can make it hard to talk about what happened.

Feeling sadness/grief/loss. Sometimes stress events include losing someone close to you or losing something that is important to you. This makes you feel sad and down.

Feeling bad about yourself. Sometimes, all this stress can make you feel really bad about yourself, like you're a bad person or that no one likes you. This makes it harder to be friendly and to have fun with others.

Having physical health problems and complaints. Stress has an effect on your body as well. People tend to get sick more often and to notice pain and discomfort more often when they have been under stress.

EDUCATION AND RELAXATION

Name: _____

1. **Did you show the "Common Reactions to Stress or Trauma" handout to your parent and talk about which problems are bothering you?**

   ❏ **Yes—How did it go?** _____

   _____

   _____

   ❏ **No—Why not?** _____

   _____

   _____

2. **When did you practice your relaxation?**

   1st time _____ **How did it go?** _____

   _____

   _____

   2nd time _____ **How did it go?** _____

   _____

   _____

   3rd time _____ **How did it go?** _____

   _____

   _____

IMAGINAL EXPOSURE TO STRESS OR TRAUMA

Individual sessions with each child should occur sometime between Group Sessions 2 and 6. Each child should have at least one session individually; in some cases, two or three individual sessions are helpful. At the end of the first individual session, decide whether or not to schedule additional sessions.

I. Explain Rationale and Answer Questions

Begin the session by explaining the rationale for stress or trauma exposure. Answer any questions that the child has. The following examples can be used:

"Have you ever eaten too much all at once and felt really full and sick afterwards? And you wish you never ate that much? Your stomach feels sick because it's got too much in it at once. That food feels like it's filling up your whole body. Your stomach has more than it can handle.

The way you think about the stressful event you went through can also feel like that— it's too much to digest at once, so it bothers you a lot. Just like with the meal, you need to "digest" it sooner or later. Even though the stress probably seems really overwhelming when you think about it now, eventually, with enough work, we can make it smaller. Today we're going to help you start to digest it, by talking about it. We'll also make a plan for how to continue digesting it for the rest of the group sessions.

By thinking about the stress or trauma where it is safe (here with me or in the group), a couple of things will happen:

AGENDA

I. **Explain Rationale and Answer Questions**

II. **Imaginal Exposure to the Stressful or Traumatic Events**

III. **Planning for Group Support**

IV. **Planning for Additional Individual Sessions**

OBJECTIVES FOR ALL INDIVIDUAL SESSIONS

1. Gather information about the trauma for use in treatment planning.
2. Reduce anxiety when remembering the trauma.
3. Plan with participant how they will work on trauma in group sessions.
4. Build rapport and trust.

SPECIAL SUPPLIES

1. Copy of the "Counseling" worksheet
2. Copy of the Fear Thermometer (Appendix B)

1. *Over time, if you work on digesting the stress or trauma, you will feel less upset each time you think about it. By the end of group you will be able to think about what happened and feel OK.*

2. *You will learn that thinking about the stress or trauma won't make you flip out or go crazy, that it's just a bad memory that can't hurt you anymore.*

3. *You will learn that you can take control of the way you feel and do something to make yourself feel better."*

II. Imaginal Exposure to the Stressful or Traumatic Events

In this part of the session, you will work with each child to remember the most stressful event or the worst traumatic event. The goals are to:

❏ Learn as much as possible about what happened so that you can plan the rest of the exposure in subsequent sessions.

❏ Begin the process of exposure to the traumatic memory.

This process may be very difficult for some children, and, so, a great deal of attention needs to be given to ensure an optimal level of involvement in the process. The ideal level of involvement is for the child to feel moderately anxious during the process but not feel overwhelmed or out of control. Techniques to increase or decrease a child's involvement are listed in **Table 3**. However, it is most important that you tailor the exercise to the individual and allow the children to have control over the process.

Common Questions

Counselors and therapists often have questions about doing this kind of work with their clients.

Am I going to retraumatize the child? Keep in mind that the stress or trauma has already occurred. Thinking about the stress or trauma is one way that we know helps children heal from the stress or trauma. As long as you work with empathy and concern for the child, you are part of the healing process. To ensure that the child does not get overly upset, you can make sure that: (1) he or she understands the reasons for doing it; (2) you follow the child's own pace and do not push too hard; (3) you provide encouragement for whatever level of engagement the child achieves, so that the process feels like a success; and (4) you anticipate problems with activities or with attending to the rest of the group. The worst-case scenario is that the child feels overwhelmed during the process and never gets the chance to finish it and to reap the benefits. Thus, it is important that children and parents are braced for the children to feel upset and are committed to returning to the group to finish the process.

Table 3: Techniques to increase or decrease involvement.

Disengaged/Numb	Overly Engaged/Upset
Ask detailed questions about sensations, emotions.	Ask neutral questions about facts.
Slow down the story ("slow motion").	Speed up the story/skip hard parts ("fast forward").
Remind member of rationale.	Touch group member (with permission). Use relaxation to calm.

Will I be able to "take it" when I hear the details of what happened? Hearing these stories can be painful, stirring up anger, despair, and fear. However, the process of being listened to is important for the child, and he or she needs to feel comfortable that you will be able to cope with it. Thus, it is important to convey empathy and caring but not to appear overwhelmed. Counselors often report their own distress (intrusive thinking, nightmares, emotional numbing) in a vicarious reaction to their patient's traumatic experiences. It is useful to seek consultation if this process or a particular stress or trauma story feels overwhelming to you.

Ask the child to pretend that the traumatic event is a movie and to "project" it onto a blank wall/desk/piece of paper. Ask him or her to describe the movie in a lot of detail, not just what is happening (the "action"), but also the setting, how people think and feel, etc. Explain that you will take some notes so that the two of you can look over the whole story and decide how to work on it when he or she is finished.

While the child is telling the story, use the guidelines in **Table 3** to help him or her manage emotional engagement with the process. Take detailed notes about what happened. Repeat the process a few times, as necessary, so that the full exercise takes about 30 minutes.

When the child is finished, go over the story together and identify different parts of it (e.g., when something specific happened, when he or she thought something in particular or felt a certain way). These parts can include things that happened after the event itself (e.g., contact with the police, visit to the doctor). Use the "Counseling" worksheet at the end of Individual Session 1 to make the list of the parts of the story. After you have created the list, ask the child

to rate each one with a number from the Fear Thermometer (Appendix B) in terms of how upsetting it feels to think about that part. (If the individual session occurs before Group Session 3, you'll have to introduce the Fear Thermometer first. See "Group Session 3" for an explanation.)

Look at the list, and pick one or two parts that evoke a moderate level of anxiety (e.g., in the 4–6 range on the Fear Thermometer) and a couple of parts that evoke a high level (e.g., 7–10). Ask the child if he or she would be willing to work on those parts in Group Sessions 8 and 9 on social problem-solving. Some guidelines for choosing parts to work on:

❑ Select parts that are long enough (more than a second or two) and rich enough that the child will be able to talk about them, imagine them, and draw pictures of them.

❑ Avoid parts that seem to evoke strong guilt reactions or anger. These emotions are less likely to be reduced through exposure alone. Instead, make sure to target those parts via cognitive therapy or normalizing in the group. There will be room to discuss these types of issues in Group Sessions 6 and 7, after the exposure exercises.

❑ Take ratings on the Fear Thermometer with a grain of salt; a 6 does not mean the same thing to everyone. Make sure to pick parts that the child will be able to tolerate but that will also offer a challenge. This may take some discussion with the child.

Examples of parts:

"When I notice that I am bleeding."

"When he says to me, 'If you tell anyone about this, I'll kill you.'"

"When I think, 'I should do something to help her.'"

Discuss the chosen parts with the child and reach an agreement about which parts he or she is willing to work on in Group Sessions 6 and 7 in each of the following ways:

1. In his or her imagination (kept completely private).

2. By drawing a picture of it (kept private or shared with group—either is fine).

3. By talking about it to the rest of the group.

Make sure that the child agrees to something in each category, but make it clear that the child can change his or her mind at any point. Fill out the "Counseling" worksheet to solidify your agreement, and keep it for your own use in the later sessions.

III. Planning for Group Support

Depending on the level of support that the children offer each other in the group, it may be helpful to explicitly plan group support. This will ensure that the children feel comfortable after they share their traumatic experiences with the group.

Begin by asking the child the following questions:

"What kind of support or feedback would you like to get from the other group members when you tell them about what happened to you?"

"Is there a particular person in the group that you want to get support or feedback from?"

"Who can you offer support to, when they tell you about what happened to them?"

"What can you tell people after they share with the group?"

"Is there anything you want to be careful not to say or do after people share?"

Help the child identify the types of support that would be helpful Then try to ensure that the child receives at least some of that support after sharing. In addition, make sure all the children understand that laughing, making fun, or ignoring other people after they share could make them feel bad, and that you will expect them to show support to all the group members.

IV. Planning for Additional Individual Sessions

Your decision about whether to schedule further sessions depends on the child's reactions in this first individual session, his or her motivation to continue, and your own judgment. If the child was distressed during the session or has suffered more than one severe trauma, a follow-up should be planned—unless the youth is extremely reluctant to do so. Explain that it's usually good to talk about these things more than once and that you'd like to schedule another time to meet alone with him or her. Elicit and address any concerns or reactions that the youth has about subsequent meetings.

Name of Child: _____

COUNSELING WORKSHEET

Part(s) of stress or trauma: **Fear Rating**

_____	_____
_____	_____
_____	_____
_____	_____
_____	_____
_____	_____
_____	_____
_____	_____
_____	_____
_____	_____
_____	_____

Part(s) that the child will work on in imagination or drawings:

_____	_____
_____	_____

Part(s) that the child will work on by talking to the group:

_____	_____
_____	_____

IMAGINAL EXPOSURE TO STRESS OR TRAUMA

I. Check-In

Begin by checking on the child's reactions to the first individual session, symptoms since then, and progress in the group. Address any worries, and reiterate the rationale presented in Individual Session 1 as needed. At times, children who are able to express emotions about trauma in the first session have trouble doing so in the second (or third) sessions. This may be in part because they are embarassed or ashamed of being upset in front of another person. So, it is quite important that you normalize any prior reactions, praise the child for his or her hard work in the last session, and make sure that the child understands the rationale for continued work.

II. Imaginal Exposure to the Traumatic Events

Conduct imaginal exposure in the same way as described in Individual Session 1. Use a new "Counseling" worksheet and repeat the process using the same trauma event or a different trauma, as needed. If there is time, ask the child to repeat the story more than one time, and make ratings on the Fear Thermometer for each repetition.

III. Planning for Group Support

Review plans for sharing in the group during Sessions 8 and 9, and adjust as needed.

AGENDA

I. Check-In
II. Imaginal Exposure to the Traumatic Events
III. Planning for Group Support
IV. Planning for an Additional Individual Session

OBJECTIVES FOR ALL INDIVIDUAL SESSIONS

1. Gather information about the trauma for use in treatment planning.
2. Reduce anxiety when remembering the trauma.
3. Plan with participant how they will work on trauma in group sessions.
4. Build rapport and trust

SPECIAL SUPPLIES

1. Copy of the "Counseling" worksheet
2. Copy of the Fear Thermometer

IV. Planning for an Additional Individual Session

As in the prior session, schedule another individual meeting if the child still appears distressed or has additional traumatic events to address.

Name of Child: _____

COUNSELING WORKSHEET

Part(s) of stress or trauma: **Fear Rating**

_____   _____

_____   _____

_____   _____

_____   _____

_____   _____

_____   _____

_____   _____

_____   _____

_____   _____

_____   _____

_____   _____

_____   _____

Part(s) that the child will work on in imagination or drawings:

_____   _____

_____   _____

_____   _____

Part(s) that the child will work on by talking to the group:

_____   _____

_____   _____

_____   _____

IMAGINAL EXPOSURE TO STRESS OR TRAUMA

I. Check-In

Begin by checking on the child's reactions to the last individual session, symptoms since then, and progress in the group. Address any worries and reiterate the rationale presented in Individual Session 1 as needed. At times, children who are able to express emotions about trauma in the first or second session have trouble doing so in the third session. This may be in part because they are embarassed or ashamed of being upset in front of another person. So, it is quite important that you normalize any prior reactions, praise the child for his or her hard work in the last session, and make sure that the child understands the rationale for continued work.

AGENDA	I. Check-In
	II. Imaginal Exposure to the Traumatic Events
	III. Planning for Group Support

OBJECTIVES FOR ALL INDIVIDUAL SESSIONS

1. Gather information about the trauma for use in treatment planning.
2. Reduce anxiety when remembering the trauma.
3. Plan with participant how they will work on trauma in group sessions.
4. Build rapport and trust

SPECIAL SUPPLIES

1. Copy of the "Counseling" worksheet
2. Copy of the Fear Thermometer

II. Imaginal Exposure to the Traumatic Events

Conduct imaginal exposure in the same way as you did during the first two individual sessions. Use a new "Counseling" worksheet and repeat the process using the same trauma event or a different trauma, as needed. If there is time, ask the child to repeat the story more than one time, and make ratings on the Fear Thermometer for each repetition.

III. Planning for Group Support

Review plans for sharing in the group during Sessions 8 and 9, and adjust as needed.

Name of Child _____

COUNSELING WORKSHEET

Part(s) of stress or trauma:

	Fear Rating

_____ _____

_____ _____

_____ _____

_____ _____

_____ _____

_____ _____

_____ _____

_____ _____

_____ _____

_____ _____

_____ _____

Part(s) that the child will work on in imagination or drawings:

_____ _____

_____ _____

_____ _____

Part(s) that the child will work on by talking to the group:

_____ _____

_____ _____

_____ _____

INTRODUCTION TO COGNITIVE THERAPY

I. Activities Review

Review group members' progress with the relaxation technique and help them solve any problems, such as:

1. **Not enough time/too noisy in the house.** Ask the group member to talk to his or her parent to figure out a way to have quiet time set aside for the relaxation exercise.

2. **Couldn't relax—kept thinking about problems.** Ask the group member to continue to practice and to make sure that he or she is doing the exercise correctly. Review the relaxation technique for the whole group if necessary. Another option is to record tapes of the instructions for group members to use at home.

3. **Felt worse/made me upset.** In some rare cases relaxation can have the opposite effect and make people feel agitated or panicky. If this seems true for an individual in the group, ask him or her to stop using the technique and to try to identify other ways to relax at home.

Ask group members if they shared the "Handout for Parents" with their parents and how that went. If group members did not complete the activity, ask them to explain why not. Use this opportunity to remind group members about the rationale:

"Though it may be embarrassing to admit that you are having any problems, these kinds of problems are really common, and your parent

AGENDA
I. Activities Review
II. Fear Thermometer
III. Thoughts and Feelings (Introduction to Cognitive Therapy)
IV. Linkage Between Thoughts and Feelings
V. Hot Seat: Combating Negative Thoughts
VI. Activities Assignment

OBJECTIVES

1. Develop common language for "level" of feelings.
2. Teach link between thoughts and feelings.
3. Build skills: Challenging negative thoughts.

SPECIAL SUPPLIES

1. Copies of Fear Thermometers (Appendix B)
2. An extra chair to use as the Hot Seat
3. Copies of the Activity Worksheets

can help you with it if he or she knows what is happening to you."

"Though it is hard to talk and think about what happened to you, part of being in this group involves digesting that experience, and the more you take advantage of opportunities to do that, the quicker you will feel better."

II. Fear Thermometer

The goal of this part of the session is to introduce a way for group members to talk about how anxious or nervous they feel in various situations:

"Today we're going to talk about feelings and thinking, but in order to do that, we need to find some way to measure how we are feeling. Who can tell me how we measure the temperature outside? We can use the same idea for

measuring how scared or upset we feel. We call it the Fear Thermometer."

Show the children the first Fear Thermometer (Appendix B). Use the other Fear Thermometers to show different levels of feelings, and ask group members to give examples of when they felt each way (not at all scared or upset; a little scared or upset; pretty scared or upset; really scared or upset). Explain that the "10" on the Fear Thermometer is kept for those times when we are completely and utterly scared and upset. Tell group members that they will be using the Fear Thermometer to tell how they feel during the rest of the group sessions. Ask each child to give their Fear Rating for right then, and make sure that they are all using the scale correctly. (Query any extreme ratings to make sure that the child is actually feeling that way.)

III. Thoughts and Feelings (Introduction to Cognitive Therapy)

The goal of this part of the session is to show that thoughts cause emotions. Begin with an example of the way thoughts can influence feelings.

For Younger Groups: [2]

"Does anyone know the story of Chicken Little? How does that go? [Fill in story details as necessary.] Chicken Little was scratching around in the barnyard, and then suddenly felt something hit him in the head. He thought to himself, 'The sky is falling!' He was so certain that the sky was falling that he ran all over the place yelling, 'The sky is falling, the sky is fall-

ing!' and everyone thought he was crazy. He was probably feeling about a '9' on the Fear Thermometer. Was the sky really falling? No. An acorn had fallen off the tree and hit Chicken Little on the head. So he had gotten all upset about nothing—just a little acorn.

"In this situation, Chicken Little's THOUGHTS got him into a lot of trouble and made him all upset. His thoughts were wrong. What would have happened if Chicken Little had thought, 'An acorn just hit me on the head!' Would he have felt as scared or upset? No, he would probably have just kept on scratching around the barnyard, without feeling scared or upset."

For Older Groups:

"Does anyone remember how the people of Europe thought the world was shaped, back before they came to America? They thought it was flat. In fact, they thought that if they sailed far enough, they'd fall off the edge of the earth and die. When the first explorers wanted to go out and find new lands, most of the Europeans thought they were crazy. They were afraid to sail too far themselves, in case they fell off the edge. But it turned out that all those people were wrong. They wasted all that time being afraid to sail around the world.

"Today, we are going to talk about the kinds of thoughts that each of you have that might be wrong and the way that you can double-check to make sure that you aren't getting upset over nothing or keeping yourself from doing things because you are afraid."

---

[2] This story was originally used to introduce the concept of thoughts determining feelings and actions in Gillham, J., Jaycox, L. H., Reivich, K. J., Seligman, M. E. P., & Silver, T. (1991). *Manual for Leaders of the Coping Skills Program for Children.* Unpublished manual. Copyright Foresight, Inc.

IV. Linkage Between Thoughts And Feelings

The goal of this part of the session is to make sure that group members understand the way in which thoughts and feelings are linked. Pick an example that is relevant to the group (use one of the group member's own problem situations, if possible) to do the following exercise:

"Different kinds of thoughts can lead to different feelings. Let's take an example.

Example 1:

"You are walking through the cafeteria at school, and a bunch of kids are laughing and looking over at you.

Example 2:

"You are waiting for your brother/sister outside of a store, and some kids come up and start to hassle you.

"What are some ways that you might feel if this happened to you? [List feelings, eliciting several different types, on the board.] So, this is interesting. We have the same situation, but it's causing all kinds of different feelings. Why is this? Let's take a look at the way that you might be thinking about this situation that would lead to the different feelings. [Fill in the possible thoughts that would lead to each of the different emotions (see **Table 4**). *Make the point that different thoughts lead to different feelings, even if the situation is exactly the same.] What might you be saying to yourself that would make you feel _____?"*

Table 4: Feelings and related thoughts.

Example 1

Feelings	Possible Thoughts
Angry	They have no right to laugh at me!
Sad	No one likes me. I'll never have good friends like that.
Embarrassed	They must think I look funny.
OK	They're just telling jokes; it's not about me.
Good	They think I'm funny and like me.

Example 2

Feelings	Possible Thoughts
Angry	They should leave me alone.
Scared	They are going to try to beat me up.
OK	They are just talking— nothing will happen.
Ashamed	Why are they picking on me? There must be something wrong with me.

V. Hot Seat: Combating Negative Thoughts [3]

The goal of this part of the session is to train group members to challenge their negative thinking. It is broken into several parts, with a bit of teaching followed by practice.

"How can you argue with negative thoughts? There are a few different ways to make sure that a thought isn't totally wrong, like Chicken Little's idea that the sky was falling.

"The first approach is to ask yourself if there are any OTHER WAYS OF THINKING (ALTERNATIVES) about this situation that make sense:

Is there another way to look at this?

Is there another reason why this would happen?

"Let's take another example [use an example from the group if possible]:

You are at home alone, and you hear a noise in the other room.

Your first thought:	Someone is breaking into the house.
Your feeling:	Scared."

Ask the children to list other possible thoughts and the feelings they evoke, and write these on the board. Make sure the alternatives make sense and are not completely irrational. As time permits, work through other examples from children's own lives on the board.

"Now it's time to PRACTICE coming up with alternative thoughts."

Group Exercise:

Introduce the Hot Seat activity, which you will use for the rest of the session. Explain that a designated chair is the "hot seat" and the person who sits in the chair practices coming up with new ways of thinking. Begin by sitting in the Hot Seat yourself. Select one child to assist you in case you get stuck and can't think of a more positive approach. Instruct the child to provide negative thoughts, one at a time. You will respond by producing alternative positive thoughts. Use the child's own examples or the one that follows:

"Consider the situation we used before:

You are home alone and you hear a noise in the other room.

What are some negative thoughts you might have? Call them out, and I'll try to come up with more positive alternatives. If I get stuck, [name of youth] will help me out."

After the exercise, review the thoughts. Identify any irrational thoughts, and point out the additional strategies for arguing with negative thoughts during the rest of this session and in Group Session 4.

Select a volunteer for the Hot Seat. Select another as "coach" to help the child in the Hot Seat contend with negative thoughts. When the child in the Hot Seat gets stuck, have the coach ask a question to help generate positive counter-thoughts. Also be prepared to serve as coach yourself to ensure that the child in the Hot Seat is supported and that

---

[3] This exercise was originally developed for use in depression prevention in children in Gillham, J., Jaycox, L. H., Reivich, K. J., Seligman, M. E. P., & Silver, T. (1991). *Manual for Leaders of the Coping Skills Program for Children.* Unpublished manual. Copyright Foresight, Inc., and was subsequently modified in a similar fashion for adolescents in Asarnow, J., Jaycox, L. H., Clarke, G., Lewinsohn, P., Hops, H., & Rohde, P. (1999a). *Stress and Your Mood: A Manual.* Los Angeles: UCLA School of Medicine.

strategies for generating positive thoughts are demonstrated. (Optional: Select some children as "recorders" to note positive and negative thoughts.)

Tell the group other situations for the Hot Seat exercise:

"You fail an important test at school."

"Your friend is supposed to call you to arrange a time to pick you up to go out, but he/she hasn't called yet."

"Your parents go out and leave you at home alone."

"You are waiting for the bus, and some older kids start to come down the block."

"Another way to work on irrational negative thoughts is to look at WHAT WILL HAPPEN (IMPLICATIONS) or to ask yourself:

> *Even if this thought is true, what's the worst thing that can happen?*

> *Even if this thought is true, what's the best thing that can happen?*

> *What will be the most likely thing to happen?*

"The trick is to look at both the positive and negative things that could happen, to make sure you aren't only thinking about the bad things that could happen. For instance, in the home-alone example, one thing you thought is 'Someone is in the other room.'

"First, ask yourself, 'Even if this thought is true, what's the WORST thing that could happen?'" [Don't spend much time on this one—move quickly to the best and most likely things.]

Elicit ideas and write them on the board:

"It could be a burglar; I could get hurt; they could take our stuff."

"Next ask yourself, 'If this thought is true, what's the BEST thing that could happen?'"

For example, maybe it's someone in your family trying to surprise you!

Elicit ideas and write them on the board.

"Finally, ask yourself, 'What will be the most likely thing to happen?'

Think, for example:

> *'I'd listen for more noises. If it's a person, I'll get out of the house and call the police or go to a neighbor's house.'"*

Elicit ideas and write them on the board.

Group Activity:

Repeat the Hot Seat activity with a new situation, using both alternatives and implications to produce positive counter-thoughts. Provide a situation to the group member in the Hot Seat, then ask these questions: "What is the worst that could happen? The best that could happen? The most likely thing to happen?" Have another group member act as coach in case the one in the Hot Seat has difficulty.

VI. Activities Assignment

Distribute copies of the Activity Worksheets that follow. Describe the assignment, which is to practice the Hot Seat thinking at home. Give group members several copies of the worksheet, and have them practice with an example before they leave the group if there is sufficient time. Try to give group members specific instructions about the kinds of situations to work on, depending on their needs. Show group members the "Hot Seat Exercise Example" to help them understand how to fill in the "Hot Seat Exercise" worksheet.

HOT SEAT ACTIVITY

Name: _____

Questions you can use to argue against negative thoughts:

Other ways to think about it—

Is there another way to look at this?

Is there another reason why this would happen?

What will happen next—

Even if this thought is true, what's the worst thing that can happen?

Even if this thought is true, what's the best thing that can happen?

What is the most likely thing to happen?

HOT SEAT EXERCISE

Name: _____

In the box, write something that happened to you that made you upset. Then write down some of the thoughts you had under "Negative Thoughts." Use the questions on the "Hot Seat Activity" worksheet to find new ways of thinking about what happened. Refer to the "Hot Seat Exercise Example" worksheet to see how to complete your own worksheet.

What happened:

Negative Thoughts:	**Hot Seat Thoughts:**

Hot Seat Exercise (Example)

What happened:
I stayed up late because I didn't want to fall asleep.

Negative Thoughts:	Hot Seat Thoughts:
If I fall asleep, I'll have nightmares.	• I don't have nightmares every night, so I might not have them tonight. • Nightmares aren't real, they can't hurt me. • I need to get some sleep for school tomorrow, even if it means I have nightmares.
If I fall asleep, something bad will happen.	• I'm safe in my house and my bed. My family is here to protect me. • If something bad happens, I'll wake up and be able to deal with it then.
Lying down in my bed makes me feel nervous.	• I can practice my relaxation if I feel nervous. • I can remind myself that I am safe. • It's OK to feel nervous for a little while; eventually I'll fall asleep.

COMBATING NEGATIVE THOUGHTS

I. Activities Review

Review the activities from the previous session. Look for the following trouble spots and correct them as needed:

1. **Didn't do any activities.** Attempt to find out why, and suggest ways to improve compliance. Ask if the group member noticed any negative thinking in the past week and to describe what it was. Ask if he challenged that negative thinking in any way. If so, praise him for work well done. If not, ask the child to try to do it right then and to ask for help from other group members if needed.

2. **Couldn't think of any Hot Seat thoughts to challenge negative thinking.** Have other group members help the child think of Hot Seat thoughts. If none are appropriate, remind the group that sometimes negative thinking is realistic and that, in those cases, it's important to try to accept the situation and figure out a way to handle it or solve the problem.

3. **The Hot Seat thoughts are unrealistic.** Sometimes group members will supply very unrealistic Hot Seat thoughts. A few thoughts like this are OK. If this happens too much, so that the exercise seems like a joke, ask the group member or the entire group if thinking this way is helpful. Remind them that they are trying to correct thinking that is wrong (go back to the Chicken Little/flat world examples), not to come up with more "wrong" thoughts.

II. Continuation of Cognitive Therapy

Pick up where you left off in the previous group session, and introduce two new ways to question negative thoughts: plan of attack and evidence for negative thoughts.

"Last time we worked on making sure that the way we THINK about things isn't too negative—that we aren't thinking like Chicken Little and thinking that the sky is falling when it is just an acorn hitting us on the head. Today we're going to find some more ways to do that.

"Another way to work on irrational negative thoughts is to look for any possible PLAN OF ATTACK. Even if your most negative thought seems true, there might be something you can do about it. Continuing with the example from the last session, what are some things you could do if you decide that the person in your house really is a burglar? Ask yourself:

'Is there anything I can do about this?'

"Remember our example from last time? You are at home alone, and you hear a noise in the other room.

Your first thought: Someone is breaking into the house.

Your feeling: Scared."

List possible plans of attack on the board, such as:

❏ Listen to see if there are more noises.

❏ Look and see what's making the noise.

❏ Go to a neighbor's house and ask them to help you check it out.

Group Activity:

Repeat the Hot Seat activity as described in Session 3 using a new situation and new alternatives, implications, and plans of attack to produce positive counter-thoughts. Then introduce "checking the facts."

"Another way to make sure you're not believing irrational negative thoughts is to try to see how true they are by CHECKING THE FACTS. We figure out if a thought is true by thinking about all the facts. Facts are things that everyone would agree are true, not feelings or guesses about things. Sometimes when we are feeling down or stressed out, we tend to focus on negative facts and ignore other facts that might lead to a more positive approach to the situation. You need to look at all of the facts in order to figure out whether your thoughts are true or not.

"The key here is to look for all kinds of facts. You need to list not only facts that say your thought is TRUE but also facts that show your thought might be FALSE. The kinds of questions you can ask yourself to find the facts are:

How do I know this is true?

Has this happened to me before?

Has this happened with other people?

"Take the example we used a minute ago. I'll list some evidence, and you tell me whether these facts show whether or not the thought 'Someone is in the other room' is TRUE or FALSE."

List facts, such as the ones that follow, under two columns: "true" and "false."

1. The cat comes running out of the room, trailing water and broken flowers. (FALSE—the cat probably knocked over a vase.)

2. There aren't any more noises for a few minutes. (FALSE)

3. You hear a couple of footsteps. (TRUE)

4. You hear a sneeze. (TRUE)

5. You are upstairs and know that all the windows and doors are locked. (FALSE)

6. Your brother sometimes comes home without you knowing it. (TRUE)

"Let's take another example. You see your good friend laughing with another person and looking over at you. You think, 'They are laughing at me. He doesn't like me anymore.'

"Let's list the kinds of facts that you could look for, ones that show this thought might be true and others that show it might be false."

Write the thought on the board and then make two columns: "true" and "false." Help group members generate facts that would fit under both columns, like the ones in **Table 5**.

Table 5: Checking the facts.

True	False
He keeps doing this day after day.	He comes over and talks to you next.
He doesn't do things with you anymore.	It turns out they were laughing about something else.
He says no when you ask him to do something.	He is still friendly with you.

Group Activity:

Repeat the Hot Seat activity with a new situation, using alternatives, implications, evidence, and a plan of attack to produce positive counter-thoughts.

III. Practice

Continue with more Hot Seat activities, using members' own examples of recent stressful situations. Have the group come up with negative thoughts related to the event. Have the child who offered the situation sit in the Hot Seat and dispute the negative thoughts. If the group has difficulty generating scenarios, supply ones that are relevant to the group members and pick anyone in the group to dispute negative thoughts.

IV. Activities Assignment

Describe the assignment, which is to practice the Hot Seat thinking at home. Give group members several copies of the worksheets, and have them practice with an example before they leave the session if there is time. Try to give group members specific instructions about the kinds of situations to work on, depending on their needs. Show group members the "Hot Seat Exercise Example" worksheet from Session 3 to help them understand how to fill in the worksheet.

HOT SEAT ACTIVITY

Name: _____

Questions you can use to argue against negative thoughts:

Other ways to think about it—

Is there another way to look at this?

Is there another reason why this would happen?

What will happen next—

Even if this thought is true, what's the worst thing that can happen?

Even if this thought is true, what's the best thing that can happen?

What is the most likely thing to happen?

Plan of attack—

Is there anything I can do about this?

Check the facts—

How do I know this is true?

Has this happened to me before?

Has this happened with other people or in other situations?

HOT SEAT EXERCISE

Name: _____

In the box, write something that happened to you that made you upset. Then write down some of the thoughts you had under "Negative Thoughts." Use the questions on the "Hot Seat Activity" worksheets to find new ways of thinking about what happened. Refer to the "Hot Seat Exercise Example" worksheet to see how to do it.

What happened:

Negative Thoughts:	Hot Seat Thoughts:

INTRODUCTION TO REAL LIFE EXPOSURE

I. Activity Review

Review the activities from the previous session. Look for the following trouble spots and correct them as indicated:

1. **Didn't do any activities.** Attempt to find out why and suggest ways to improve compliance. Ask if the group member noticed any negative thinking during the past week and to describe it. Ask if she challenged that negative thinking in any way. If so, praise her for work well done. If not, ask the child to try to do it right then and ask for help from other group members if needed.

2. **Couldn't think of any Hot Seat thoughts to challenge negative thinking.** Have other group members help the child think of Hot Seat thoughts that could challenge negative thinking. If none are appropriate, remind the group that sometimes negative thinking is realistic and that, in those cases, it's important to try to accept the situation and figure out a way to handle it or solve the problem (though this kind of response is also an "Is there anything I can do?" response).

3. **The Hot Seat thoughts are unrealistic.** Sometimes group members will supply very unrealistic Hot Seat thoughts. A few thoughts like this are OK. If this happens too much, so that the exercise seems like a joke, ask the group member or the entire group if thinking this way is helpful. Remind them that they are trying to correct thinking that is wrong

	I. Activities Review
	II. Avoidance and Coping (Introduction to Real Life Exposure)
AGENDA	III. Construction of Fear Hierarchy
	IV. Alternative Coping Strategies
	V. Activities Assignment

OBJECTIVES

1. Identify trauma-related avoidance.
2. Plan to decrease avoidance.
3. Plan to decrease anxiety through approaching trauma reminders.
4. Build skills: Thought stopping, distraction, positive imagery.

SPECIAL SUPPLIES

1. Copies of the Activity worksheets

(go back to the Chicken Little/flat world examples), not to come up with more "wrong" thoughts.

II. Avoidance and Coping (Introduction to Real Life Exposure)

The goal of this part of the session is to introduce the idea that avoidance is one form of coping with anxiety-provoking events, but that it usually creates more problems than it solves. Begin with an example (from the group, if possible) of an anxiety-provoking event:

"Let's take an example. What kinds of things make you really nervous or afraid? (Possible examples: the first day at school, a big test at school, asking someone out for a date, performing something in front of an audience, going somewhere new alone, etc.). Have you ever felt

so nervous about something that you wished you could get away with skipping it altogether? Did you ever try to do that—avoid doing something? This is a common way to handle stress: try to avoid it. But what happens when you avoid something? Does the problem go away? Do you ever miss out on things you want to happen because you avoid something? [Discuss their experiences.]

"There's another problem with avoiding things. The more you avoid something, the scarier that thing seems. [Use a relevant example here or the one that follows.] Let's say you are really nervous about starting in a new school. You wish you didn't have to go there at all. You feel sick; you are all tense.

"If you stayed home the first day, how do you think you'd feel the second day? Would you feel less nervous, the same, or more nervous? [Make the point that they'd probably feel even more nervous, since they'd be one day behind, others would know each other, etc.]

"What if you went ahead and went to school on that first day, even though you were nervous. How would you feel the second day?" [Make the point that they would probably feel less nervous as each day went on, as long as nothing bad happened.]

Use other examples, as necessary, until the group members are convinced that repeated exposure to feared events will make them less afraid. Possible examples include: performances (sports, dance, music), speaking in class, going to unfamiliar places, and trying new things.

"In this group, we're going to start to work on things that make us nervous or upset, and we're going to do them again and again until we feel OK."

III. Construction of Fear Hierarchy

The goal of this part of the session is to build a list of situations that make each group member feel anxious or upset, and then to rank them in terms of how much anxiety each situation causes. Use the Activity worksheets that follow. Group members will need help along the way, since stress or trauma survivors are often unaware of these types of situations (especially if they are avoiding them effectively).

"Let's begin by making a list of all the kinds of situations that make you nervous or upset, especially ones that started to make you feel upset because they remind you of the stresses or traumas you went through. Put down everything you can think of while we talk; it doesn't mean that you'll have to work on it—that will be up to you to decide later. But it's important to get down everything you can think of."

Use the following questions to guide the activity. Have group members offer examples. Circulate around the room to see how group members are doing as you ask the questions, taking 15–20 minutes for the activity. There are several important things to discuss with group members as they build their lists using the worksheet:

1. The situations on the list need to be SAFE. List only things that the children should feel comfortable doing. Examples of situations that would not work are: being exposed to violence in person, doing anything dangerous, and being in an unsafe environment (e.g., out alone in a deserted area at night). If group members list such things, tell them that those things are supposed to make people nervous, because they are dangerous. You are trying to help them feel less nervous in situations in which they are supposed to feel OK. Tell them that in a few minutes you will introduce

ways to calm down when these things happen.

2. Some situations are designed to make people feel nervous or excited, and are hard to work on. These include watching scary movies and riding roller coasters. Explain to the children that part of the fun of these is to feel scared, and make sure that they really want to work on those things.

3. The lists should include things that the children are avoiding. They may not be sure how anxious they would be in these situations. For these situations, ask them to guess how nervous or upset the thing or situation would make them.

Questions:

❑ *"Are there any things that you used to do regularly that you stopped doing after the stress or trauma you went through? Examples: going to places that remind you of what happened, doing things like you were doing when the stress or trauma happened."*

❑ *"Have you started avoiding things like being alone in certain places, being in the dark, or sleeping by yourself?"*

❑ *"Do you avoid talking to people about what happened? Is there anyone that you'd like to be able to talk to about it?"*

❑ *"Do you avoid reading things or watching certain TV programs that would remind you about what happened?"*

❑ *"Do you avoid certain objects that would make you nervous or upset because they were there when it happened?"*

After group members have created their lists, use the Fear Thermometer (Appendix B) to rate each item for the anxiety it would cause:

"Now let's figure out how much each of the things on your list would bother you if you did it today. If you did it recently, you can write

down how much it bothered you then. Use the Fear Thermometer [show graphic] to rate each one. If it wouldn't bother you very much, give it a low number, like a 1 or 2 or 3. If it would bother you a whole lot, give it a high number like a 7 or 8 or 9."

Work individually with group members to identify items on the list that are likely to be beneficial to work on. Do not include any items that might pose a danger to the group member (either because the situation itself poses risks or because the group member will lack the parental supervision necessary to make the assignment work). The first priority is safety; the second priority is to assure that the group member has a high likelihood of decreasing anxiety, rather than feeling overwhelmed or out of control. Examples of good exercises include the following, with parental supervision in place: crossing roads at traffic lights, sleeping with the lights off or with the door closed, looking at pictures that remind them of the trauma, visiting a location that is similar to one in which the trauma occurred (if safe, such as a shopping mall, school, or other public place). See the full discussion of the activities assignment in Section V.

IV. Alternative Coping Strategies

Begin by asking the group what they can do if they feel anxious or nervous when they are in some way reminded of the trauma (such as the things or situations on their lists). After some group discussion, practice the following techniques:

❑ **Thought Stopping.** Begin by asking the group to think about the traumas that they experienced. Ask them to think about what happened; what it looked like; what they heard, saw, smelled, tasted, thought about, felt. Facilitate this imaginative process for a minute or so, and then say,

"STOP!" loudly to distract the group. Ask them what they are thinking about now. Most will tell you that they are thinking about you, or the other group members, or about nothing at all. Explain that this is thought stopping. Encourage them to talk about ways they can use this technique when upsetting thoughts are bothering them.

❑ **Distraction.** Next discuss distraction. Ask for examples from the group members about how they distract themselves when they are upset. These can include getting involved in a book or TV program, playing games, exercising, or talking to friends.

❑ **Positive Imagery.** Another way to reduce anxiety is to change negative images into positive ones, or to replace negative thoughts and images with positive ones. Have group members tell you things that they love to do or really great things that happened to them. Examples include lying on the beach, taking a warm bath, hiking in the mountains, riding a bike, or some particularly meaningful event. Ask group members to close their eyes and imagine this scene or event, helping them build the image by asking questions like, "How do you feel? What are you doing? What is going on around you? What do you hear? What do you smell or taste?"

❑ **Relaxation.** Remind group members of the relaxation exercise taught in Group Session 2, and review or practice as a group if necessary.

Explain that if they practice a technique enough, they will be able to call it up in times of stress to reduce anxiety. Have each group member pick one or two techniques to practice.

V. Activities Assignment

> **Parent phone call:**
>
> Call parents at this point to gain their help and support in the real life exposures techniques and to remind them of what to expect. Inform group members before you call.

Work with group members individually to identify specific things from their lists (the first Activity worksheet). Pick items on the list that seem manageable and that have a rating of 4 or less.

Distribute copies of the Assignment worksheet and ask the children to pick two things to practice from their lists and to write them on the lines below "This week, I am going to:" on the worksheet. After they write down the two things, ask them to talk to you about when and where they are going to do them. Have them write this information in the boxes on their worksheets. Ask them how they will explain the activity to their parents. Be sure to assess the safety of the situations, and help the children make adjustments as necessary to ensure they are supported by parents and will be safe during the activity. Show the children how to mark the "Fear Thermometer Rating" boxes with the levels from their Fear Thermometers before and after the activity, and at its highest level. Show the children how to fill in the boxes each time they do the activity.

The success of behavioral exposure is your responsibility, even though the group members work on these things at home, between sessions. This means that it is up to you to help group members pick reasonable assignments, plan them in enough detail so that they know exactly what to do, and anticipate and discuss potential problems ahead of time. For instance, if a group member chooses sleeping alone with the lights off but shares a room with a sibling, you will have to help him or her plan how to accomplish this. You may find it necessary to involve parents directly in order to get their assistance and support in creating exercises for group members.

In addition to logistic constraints, help group members anticipate negative thoughts that might interfere with the activity. For instance, ask, "When you first start to do this, what negative thoughts might come into your head?" Have them develop Hot Seat thoughts in advance and write them down so that they can readily access the counter-thought when needed.

Safety is a key issue. Make sure that the group members are planning assignments that will not expose them to any real danger over and above what they experience on a daily basis. For instance, pick assignments that fit into group members' existing schedule and activities. If in doubt, consult with parents about particular assignments. But beware that parents have their own trauma histories and avoidance techniques, and may

be overly protective because of their own fears. If this appears to be the case, reiterate the rationale for these techniques and suggest that the parent engage in the exercises with the child if appropriate.

The best assignments for the first week are ones that can be done repetitively (e.g., are at home or close to home, or are part of the group member's normal schedule) and evoke moderate but manageable anxiety (around a 4 on the Fear Thermometer). Look for these, and if they aren't on the list already, add some that will make this first try a successful one.

You may notice that, when you begin to assign specific activities, group members get nervous. Be sure to conduct the assignment as a collaborative process so that group members feel in control of the process. Reiterate the rationale and examples when necessary. Remind the group members that this work will make them feel better and able to do a whole range of activities.

LIST OF THINGS THAT MAKE ME FEEL NERVOUS OR AFRAID OR THAT I AVOID

Name: _____

Situation	Fear Rating
Example: Sleeping alone at night	4

FACING YOUR FEARS

1) **Choose something from the list that you are sure you can manage, with a rating of no more than 4 for your first try.**

2) **Figure out when and where you can try to do the thing you chose.**

   – You need to do it over and over again, not just once or twice.

   – You need to be able to do it SAFELY:

   • Don't do anything that will put you in danger.

   • Don't do anything without telling someone first.

3) **Tell a parent what you are going to do. Make sure your parent understands what you plan and can help you with it, if you need help.**

4) **When you do it, stick with it no matter how nervous you feel. Keep at it until you begin to feel a little bit less nervous or upset. You can use the relaxation technique if you need it. You might need to stick with it for a long time, up to an hour, before you start to feel better. If you don't feel better after an hour, make sure to try it again and again. Eventually, with enough practice, you'll start to feel more comfortable.**

5) **Fill out the Assignment worksheet and show how you felt on the Fear Thermometer before and after each time you did it. Also, tell what your highest level on the Fear Thermometer was. Talk to your group leader if you don't see any improvement.**

6) **If you feel very anxious, use one of the following skills to help yourself feel better:**

   • Thought stopping.

   • Distraction.

   • Positive images.

   • Relaxation.

ASSIGNMENT

Name: _____

This week, I am going to:

1) _____

This shows you how I felt when I did it:

When / Where?	Fear Thermometer Rating		
	Before	After	Highest
1st time			
2nd time			
3rd time			
4th time			
5th time			

2) _____

This shows you how I felt when I did it:

When / Where?	Fear Thermometer Rating		
	Before	After	Highest
1st time			
2nd time			
3rd time			
4th time			
5th time			

EXPOSURE TO STRESS OR TRAUMA MEMORY

I. Activities Review

Review children's progress with the real life exposure to stress or trauma. Highlight the fact that, if practiced enough, anxiety or upset decreases. Give a few examples of this in the group. Look for the following problems, and discuss potential solutions. As you review success with the assignment, note other fears from the "List of Things That Make Me Feel Nervous" worksheet that would be appropriate for each group member so that the activity at the end of Session 6 is easier.

1. **Didn't do the activities.** Explore why and look for avoidance. Use this opportunity to review negative thoughts and practice Hot Seat exercises if possible (e.g., ask "When it was time to do the activity, what thought popped into your head that made you decide not to do it?").

2. **Started to do it, but felt upset and cut it short.** Commend group member on his courage, but point out that this won't help him feel better. Reiterate the assignment and the need to stick with it until anxiety decreases. Talk about ways to redo the assignment in the coming week with more support or using an easier fear.

3. **Logistics interfered.** Problem-solve with the group to figure out ways to get around barriers to the activities assignment.

4. **Did it but never felt upset.** This could mean that the group member is mak-

<table>
<tr><td rowspan="4">**AGENDA**</td><td>I.   **Activity Review**</td></tr>
<tr><td>II.   **Exposure to Trauma Memory Through Imagination and Drawing/Writing**</td></tr>
<tr><td>III.   **Providing Closure to the Exposure**</td></tr>
<tr><td>IV.   **Activities Assignment**</td></tr>
</table>

OBJECTIVES

1. Decrease anxiety when remembering trauma.
2. Help children "process" the traumatic event.
3. Build peer support and reduce stigma.

SPECIAL SUPPLIES

1. Paper for drawing or lined paper for writing narratives
2. Drawing and writing implements
3. Copies of the Activity Worksheets

ing progress or avoiding the assignment somehow (e.g., using some kind of "security blanket" or safety net that makes the situation somehow not count). Examples of this include having someone there for support, doing it at a certain time of day, etc. Explore if there was anything special that made him or her feel OK. If so, consider asking the group member to remove that part of the experience to make the assignment more challenging next time. Remember that the goal is to eliminate all stress- or trauma-related avoidance. Unless the group member is likely to encounter a particular situation in his or her real life, it is not necessary to work on it.

5. **Started to feel unsafe because something happened.** If something happened that was potentially dangerous (or that would cause anxiety in anyone who was there), then this reaction is normal and healthy. Congratulate group members on their good judgment

in detecting real danger. Discuss ways to plan the next assignment to avoid any real danger and involve the group in solving this problem. Remind group members that you are working on stress- or trauma-related distress, not trying to make sure they never feel upset again.

II. Exposure to Trauma Memory Through Imagination and Drawing/Writing

The goal of this part of the session is to continue exposure to the memory of the stress or trauma in a group format. Depending on how the individual encounters went, the level of symptoms among group members, and the nature of the traumas, specific techniques are chosen for use in this and the next session. The techniques include:

1. **Leading children in imagining the stress or trauma scenes chosen in the individual sessions.** This is a good warm-up exercise for the drawing/writing exercises. For instance, review with each child briefly the scene that was agreed upon in the individual sessions. Then say to the group:

   "Now we are going to each imagine the part of the event that we just talked about. Please lean back in your chair and close your eyes. Try to picture that part of what happened to you. As I talk, imagine the things I ask you about. I'll be talking with each of you from time to time, so try not to let it distract you when you hear me talking to others. I'll be asking some questions to help you imagine it, but do not answer me aloud. [Talk slowly and ask the following questions. Monitor the group and stop by to check in with group members as needed, either to make sure they are doing the exercise or to help keep them from getting overly upset.] *Who is in your picture?*

   What is happening? What does it look like? How do you feel as this is happening? What are you thinking? Doing?

   "What are the smells? Sounds? Tastes? Feelings of things that you touch? What happens next? How do you feel as this is happening? What are you thinking? Doing?"

   Optional: A relaxation exercise may be helpful if group members seem shaken at the end of the exercise.

2. **Drawing pictures (younger/less verbal children) or writing the narrative of the stress or traumatic event.** This allows for creative expression of the stress or trauma memory and can be especially useful if the memory has just been "primed" by the imagination exercise. These drawings/narratives can be shared with the group or kept private. Ask group members to describe their pictures or to read their narratives aloud. Then ask other group members to offer support. Be careful to make sure that the other group members do not make judgmental comments or ignore the disclosure. If any of this does occur, process it by reviewing common reactions to stress or trauma and normalizing other group members' reactions. Let group members know ahead of time that you do not want them to provide too much detail to the other group members about what happened, because it's hard for others to hear so many stories. Instead, ask them to focus more on the details of how they felt and what they were thinking at the time. Warn them that you may stop them if you feel like they are giving too much detail.

3. **Telling the group about specific parts of the stress or traumatic event.** This can be more upsetting but also most

helpful. Use this technique carefully with events that children are able to process already and won't overwhelm other group members. This technique is less structured than sharing the drawings or narratives, and may be most appropriate in groups of older children. Leave time for processing the disclosures. Before using this technique, coach group members that they will need to give support after disclosures, not judgments or withdrawal. Let group members know ahead of time that you do not want them to provide too much detail to the other group members about what happened, because it's hard for others to hear so many stories. Instead, ask them to focus on the details of how they felt and what they were thinking at the time. Warn them that you may stop them if you feel like they are giving too much detail.

Use information from the individual sessions to encourage group members to offer support to each other. Before you begin, remind them of the importance of being supportive. Model offering supportive statements yourself first, then ask group members to say something as well. Do not allow group members to ignore or make fun of each other.

If the individual session(s) and assignments went well, and a group member appears to have worked through some of the distress related to the trauma, consider assigning work on a second traumatic event in addition to the first. You may also include this as part of the group member's assignment if you believe he or she would be able to work on it successfully.

During this part of the session, take the time to reinforce skills already learned by group members. For instance, use the Hot Seat to counteract particularly difficult thoughts (af-

ter the exercise is over.) You might introduce this idea by saying:

"I noticed that during the trauma you thought, 'Its all my fault.' When you think about it right now, how true do you think that is? [If group member still thinks it's true, continue.] Remember when we worked on Hot Seat thoughts? Is there a Hot Seat thought that is more realistic that might work better for this situation?"

If a group member has difficulty generating an alternative thought, ask for help from the group until a more realistic thought is offered.

III. Providing Closure to the Exposure

The goal of this part of the session is to provide closure to the exercise by leading a discussion of what was helpful. Ask the following questions of group members:

- ❑ *"How did it feel to spend time thinking about what happened? Was it better or worse than you expected?"*
- ❑ *"How did it feel to share what happened to you with the group? Was it better or worse than you expected?"*
- ❑ *"What did other group members say to you that was helpful?"*
- ❑ *"How do you think it will feel the next time you think about/talk about what happened to you?"*
- ❑ *"What do you want to do in the next session to make this a better experience for you?"*

IV. Activities Assignment

Use the Assignment—Part 1" worksheet to assign both real life exposures and stress or trauma memory work (use additional copies if necessary). Assign activities individually to group members, using one of the following options to continue exposure:

1. Have group members finish the drawings or narratives they began in Part II. (These should be about parts of an event that need more work than they received in the group session.) Make specific suggestions about parts to focus on.

2. Ask the group members to spend time looking at the pictures or reading the stories. Ask them to spend time imagining the traumatic part of the story several times.

3. Continue with real life exposure assignments using the "Assignment—Part 1" worksheet.

4. Practice the Hot Seat exercise, using the "Assignment—Part 2" worksheet.

ASSIGNMENT – PART 1

Name: _____

This week, I am going to:

1) _____

This shows you how I felt when I did it:

	When / Where?	Before	After	Highest
1st time				
2nd time				
3rd time				
4th time				
5th time				

Fear Thermometer Rating

2) _____

This shows you how I felt when I did it:

	When / Where?	Before	After	Highest
1st time				
2nd time				
3rd time				
4th time				
5th time				

Fear Thermometer Rating

ASSIGNMENT – PART 2: HOT SEAT THOUGHTS

Name: _____

In the box, write something that happened to you that made you upset. Then write down some of the thoughts you had under "Negative Thoughts."

> **What happened:**
>
>
>
>
>

Negative Thoughts:	**Hot Seat Thoughts:**
_____	_____
_____	_____
_____	_____
_____	_____
_____	_____
_____	_____
_____	_____
_____	_____
_____	_____
_____	_____

EXPOSURE TO STRESS OR TRAUMA MEMORY

I. Activities Review

Review the activities with group members, asking how they felt when they did imaginal exercises, drawing, or writing about the stresses or traumas. Look for the following trouble spots and correct them as indicated:

1. **Didn't do any activities.** Explore reasons for this. Was it fear? Reluctance to feel upset? Wanting to avoid thinking about the stress or trauma? If so, review the rationale for treatment. If possible, engage other group members to help you convince the child that this work is valuable, though painful. Try to come up with a relevant analogy (e.g., "no pain, no gain") that will motivate the child. Remind him or her that this work is time-limited, that he or she will not need to do it anymore once the group is over. Use this opportunity to review negative thoughts and practice Hot Seat exercises if possible (e.g., "When it was time to do the activities, what thoughts popped into your head that made you decide not to do them?").

2. **Didn't have time/privacy/etc.** Work on logistic barriers to activity completion with group members to ensure success in the coming week. Gently explore other possible reasons for resistance, as listed in #1.

3. **Didn't bother me/wasn't upsetting.** This could either mean progress or avoidance. Explore whether or not the group member did the exercise fully and was working on the painful parts

of the memory. If it seems that he or she did it correctly, it is possible that the memory just isn't as painful as expected. If the exercise wasn't done correctly, gently confront avoidance and make it a point to work on those areas in the rest of the session.

4. **Felt awful/too upsetting.** Reframe this as positive and courageous work on the problem. Remind the group member that it takes time before the memory becomes less upsetting but that he or she is doing what needs to be done in order to feel better. Closely monitor exposure in the rest of the session, and help the group member modulate emotions (e.g., slow down with relaxation) during the exercise so that he or she can do this at home as well.

Be sure to review the other assignments as well, checking in on real life exposure and Hot Seat practice.

II. Exposure to Trauma Memory Through Imagination and Drawing/Writing

Based on a group member's work in the previous session and on the activities, it may be necessary to modify the goals for exposure that were formulated in the individual session. In this part of the session, challenge the group member to work on a more difficult part of the stress or trauma memory, but only if he or she has been successful in the previous exercises. Otherwise, you may choose to repeat an earlier exercise and perhaps to modify it to make it more useful. As in the last session, the options include:

1. **Leading children in imagining the stress or trauma scenes chosen in the individual sessions.** This is a good warm-up exercise for the drawing/writing exercises. For instance, review with each child briefly the scene that was agreed upon in the individual session. Then say to the group:

   "Now we are going to each imagine the part of the event that we just talked about. Please lean back in your chair and close your eyes. Try to picture that part of what happened to you. As I talk, imagine the things I ask you about. I'll be talking with each of you from time to time, so try not to let it distract you when you hear me talking to others. [Talk slowly and ask the following questions. Monitor the group and stop by to check in with group members as needed, either to make sure they are doing the exercise or to help keep them from getting overly upset.] *Who is in your picture? What is happening? What does it look like? How do you feel as this is happening? What are you thinking? Doing?*

   "What are the smells? Sounds? Tastes? Feelings of things that you touch? What happens next? How do you feel as this is happening? What are you thinking? Doing?"

   Optional: A relaxation exercise may be helpful if group members seem shaken at the end of the exercise.

2. **Drawing pictures (younger/less verbal children) or writing the narrative of the traumatic event.** This allows for creative expression of the stress or trauma memory, and can be especially useful if the memory has just been "primed" by the imagination exercise. These drawings/narratives can be shared with the group or kept private. Ask group members to describe their pictures or to read their narratives aloud. Then ask other group members to offer support. Be careful to make sure that the other group members do not make judgmental comments or ignore the disclosure. If any of this does occur, process it by reviewing common reactions to stress or trauma and normalizing other group members' reactions. Let group members know ahead of time that you do not want them to provide too much detail to the other group members about what happened, because it's hard for others to hear so many stories. Instead, ask them to focus more on the details of how they felt and what they were thinking at the time. Warn them that you may stop them if you feel like they are giving too much detail.

3. **Telling the group about specific parts of the stress or traumatic event.** This can be more upsetting but also most helpful. Use this technique carefully with events that children are able to process already and won't overwhelm

other group members, perhaps after imagination exercise. This technique is less structured than sharing the drawings or narratives, and may be most appropriate in groups of older children. Leave time for processing the disclosures. Coach group members, before using this technique, that they will need to give support after disclosures, not judgments or withdrawal. Let group members know ahead of time that you do not want them to provide too much detail to the other group members about what happened, because it's hard for others to hear so many stories. Instead, ask them to focus on the details of how they felt and what they were thinking at the time. Warn them that you may stop them if you feel like they are giving too much detail.

As in the last session, it may be appropriate to turn to a second or even a third traumatic event if the group member has made sufficient progress on the one that was deemed the most upsetting.

During this part of the session, take the time to reinforce skills already learned by group members. For instance, use the Hot Seat to counteract particularly difficult thoughts (when the exercise is over). You might introduce this idea by saying:

"I noticed that during the trauma you thought, 'It's all my fault.' When you think about it right now, how true do you think that is? [If group member still thinks it's true, continue.] Remember when we worked on Hot Seat thoughts? Is there a Hot Seat thought that is more realistic that might work better for this situation?"

If a group member has difficulty generating an alternative thought, ask for help from the group until a more realistic thought is offered.

III. Providing Closure to the Exposure

The goal of this part of the session is to provide closure to the exercise by leading a discussion of what was helpful in the exercise. Ask the following questions of group members:

- ❏ *"How did it feel to spend time thinking about what happened? Was it better or worse than you expected?"*
- ❏ *"How did it feel to share what happened to you with the group? Was it better or worse than you expected?"*
- ❏ *"What did other group members say to you that was helpful?"*
- ❏ *"How do you think it will feel the next time you think about/talk about what happened to you?"*
- ❏ *"What do you want to do in the future to keep working on this problem?"*

IV. Activities Assignment

Use the Activity Worksheets that follow to assign both real life exposures and stress or trauma memory work (use additional copies if necessary). Assign activities individually to group members, using one of the following options to continue exposure:

1. Have group members finish the drawings or narratives they began in Part II. These should be about parts of the events that need more work than they received in the group session. Make specific suggestions about parts to focus on.

2. Ask the group members to spend time looking at the pictures or reading the stories. Ask them to spend time imagining the traumatic part of the story several times.

3. Continue real life exposure assignments using the "Assignment—Part 1" worksheet.

4. Practice the Hot Seat exercise, using the "Assignment—Part 2" worksheet.

ASSIGNMENT – PART 1

Name: _____

This week, I am going to:

1) _____

This shows you how I felt when I did it:

Fear Thermometer Rating

	When / Where?	Before	After	Highest
1st time				
2nd time				
3rd time				
4th time				
5th time				

2) _____

This shows you how I felt when I did it:

Fear Thermometer Rating

	When / Where?	Before	After	Highest
1st time				
2nd time				
3rd time				
4th time				
5th time				

ASSIGNMENT – PART 2

Name: _____

In the box, write something that happened to you that made you upset. Then write down some of the thoughts you had under "Negative Thoughts."

What happened:

Negative Thoughts:	Hot Seat Thoughts:
_____	_____
_____	_____
_____	_____
_____	_____
_____	_____
_____	_____
_____	_____
_____	_____
_____	_____
_____	_____

INTRODUCTION TO SOCIAL PROBLEM-SOLVING

I. Activities Review

Review the activities with group members, as you did in the last session. Ask how they felt when they did imaginal exercises, drawing, or writing about the stress or trauma. Look for the following trouble spots and correct them as indicated.

1. **Didn't do any activities.** Explore reasons for this. Was it fear? Reluctance to feel upset? Wanting to avoid thinking about the stress or trauma? If so, review the rationale for treatment. If possible, engage other group members to help you convince the child that this work is valuable, though painful. Try to come up with a relevant analogy (e.g., "no pain, no gain") that will motivate the child. Remind him or her that avoidance makes people get more anxious and upset about things over time. Use this opportunity to review negative thoughts and practice Hot Seat activities if possible (e.g., "When it was time to do the activities, what thoughts popped into your head that made you decide not to do them?").

2. **Didn't have time/privacy/etc.** Work on logistic barriers to activity completion with group members to ensure success in the coming week. Gently explore other possible reasons for resistance, as listed in #1.

3. **Didn't bother me/wasn't upsetting.** This could either mean progress or avoidance. Explore whether or not the group member did the exercise fully and was working on the painful parts of the memory. If it seems that he or she did it correctly, it is possible that the memory just isn't as painful as expected. If the exercise wasn't done correctly, gently confront avoidance and remind group members that avoidance will only make them feel more anxious or upset over time.

4. **Felt awful/too upsetting.** Reframe this as positive and courageous work on the problem. Remind the group member that it takes time before the memory becomes less upsetting but that he or she is doing what needs to be done in order to feel better. Be attentive to unfinished business in discussing continued work and relapse prevention. Consider continuing individual therapy with the group member, if necessary, until the distress decreases.

AGENDA

I. Activities Review
II. Introduction to Social Problem-Solving
III. Link Between Negative Thoughts and Actions
IV. Brainstorming Solutions
V. Decision Making: Pros and Cons
VI. Activities Assignment

OBJECTIVES

1. Teach link between thoughts and actions.
2. Build skills: Social problem-solving.
3. Help children deal with real life problems.

SPECIAL SUPPLIES

1. Copies of the Activity Worksheets

Be sure to review the other assignments as well, checking in on real life exposure and Hot Seat practice.

II. Introduction to Social Problem-Solving[1]

The purpose of this part of the session is to briefly introduce the idea that solving problems with other people takes practice. Begin by asking group members to list conflicts or problems they have with friends or family members; write these on the board. As much as possible, draw from this list of problems during the rest of the session. In choosing examples for the group, consider the types of symptoms they are expressing and how well they work together within the group. Two types of examples are possible: (1) a general example drawing on common peer or family problems (but about anxiety and/or avoidance); and (2) a stress- or trauma-focused example relating to social situations (e.g., disclosure about abuse, avoidance that interferes with friendships). Both examples are shown in Section III. Introduce social problem-solving as follows:

"Sometimes people think they are upset because they have 'real problems' and 'anyone who had these problems would be upset.'

"If you feel this way, you usually think you have to solve the problem in order to feel better. But that's not true. You DO have some control over feeling better.

"There are four parts to every problem:

1. *Physical (objective, measurable) events.*

2. *How others think and act.*

3. *How you think.*

4. *How you act or what you do.*

We can work today on how you think about things and how you act on them."

III. Link Between Negative Thoughts and Actions

Continuing with social problem-solving, this part of the session reviews the ways in which thoughts influence behavior with friends and family members. Make the point that different thoughts lead to different actions and that one way to change the way we act with friends and family is to check our thinking about what happened.

Example 1 (General):

"Tom's friends are all going to a dance at school, and all of them have asked dates. Tom is the only one who hasn't asked anyone yet. Tom is afraid that the person he likes, Yolanda, won't want to go with him, so he's been avoiding asking her. He is walking down the hall and sees Yolanda talking to a guy in his class, and he thinks, 'She's going to the dance with him.' So he turns the corner to avoid her and goes straight home from school."

"In this example, what did Tom think? What did he do? [Write thoughts and actions in two columns on the board as in **Table 6**.] *You can see that what Tom did made complete sense, given what he thought. Who can tell me some other ways to think about this problem?"* [List several other thoughts as in **Table 7**, using Hot Seat questions if necessary. Then review each thought, and say what Tom would do if he was thinking that way.]

---

[1] This introduction about the "healthy management of reality" is derived from Muñoz, R. F., & Miranda, J. (1986). *Group Therapy Manual for Cognitive-Behavioral Treatment of Depression.* San Francisco General Hospital, Depression Clinic. (Activities – Session 4), and, as modified for adolescents, in Asarnow, J., Jaycox, L. H., Clarke, G., Lewinsohn, P., Hops, H., & Rohde, P. (1999a). *Stress and Your Mood: A Manual.* Los Angeles: UCLA School of Medicine.

Table 6: Tom's possible thoughts and actions.

Thoughts	Actions
She's going to the dance with him.	NOT ask her out—go home.
She's telling him that she likes ME.	Go up now and ask her out.

Table 7: More possible thoughts and actions of Tom.

Thoughts	Actions
They are talking about school.	Find her later and ask her out.
Maybe she's going to the dance with him.	Ask around and see if that's true.
If she says no, I can ask someone else.	Ask her first, then someone else.

Example 2 (Trauma-Related):

"You tell one friend about what happened to you, and she doesn't say much to you and leaves a little while later. You go to school the next day, and your friend is talking with a group of other kids. You think your friend is telling them what happened to you, and feel really mad and upset. You avoid her, and hang up on your friend when she calls you at home that night.

"In this example, what did you think? What did you do? [Write thoughts and actions in two columns on the board as in Table 8.] You can see that what you did made complete sense, given what you thought. Who can tell me some other ways to think about this problem?" [List several other thoughts on the board as in Table 9, using Hot Seat questions if necessary. Then review each thought, and say what you would do if you were thinking this way.]

Table 8: Possible thoughts and actions in Example 2.

Thoughts	Actions
She told everyone what happened to me.	Avoid everyone.
They all feel sorry for me.	Get some sympathy from them.
They all think I'm a reject.	Avoid everyone.

Table 9: More possible thoughts and actions in Example 2.

Thoughts	Actions
She's busy with them now, but she wouldn't tell them about me.	Catch up with her later.
It's going to take her some time to realize what I went through, then she'll be nice to me again.	Let it go for now, but talk to her when she calls.
She's not a good friend after all.	Realize she isn't trustworthy, but try to talk to someone else about it another time.

To summarize, make the point that different thoughts about a problem will lead to doing things differently to handle the problem. So, it is important to make sure that your thinking is accurate before you decide what to do.

IV. Brainstorming Solutions

The goal of this part of the session is to practice generating lots of solutions to real life problems, so that group members aren't "locked in" to one type of response (often based on faulty thinking). This part of the session is especially important for those group members who tend to act impulsively. It helps them slow down the thought process and give themselves more options for how to act. Encourage group members to be creative but also to include appropriate behaviors as much as possible. Follow through with the examples used in Section III, or use a new example based on issues that have come up. To break up the didactic presentation, divide the group into two teams and have them work on the same example. Tell the group that the team that comes up with the most possible actions will win the competition. Then reconvene as a group and review all the possibilities generated.

Example 1 (General):

"What are some different things that Tom could do in this situation?

"Let's list them on the board:

- *Ask her if she's going to the dance, and if not, ask her out.*

- *Ask her friends if she's going to the dance.*

- *If she's going to the dance, think of someone else to ask.*

- *Decide not to go to the dance, but make some other plans."*

Example 2 (Trauma-Related):

"What are some different things that you could do in this situation?

"Let's list them on the board:

- *Ask your friend if she told others.*

- *If she did tell others, explain to her how you feel about it.*

- *Try to find friends who are more trustworthy.*

- *Shake it off—it doesn't matter if they know what happened."*

V. Decision Making: Pros and Cons

The goal of this part of the session is to evaluate the possible actions the children are considering. For younger groups, use the terminology "pluses and minuses" and for older groups "pros and cons." Pick one of the favorite actions that go with the two examples given in Section III, and write it on the board, then make two columns labeled "pluses" or "pros" and "minuses" or "cons." Divide the group into two teams, and ask them to generate reasons why the favorite action would be a good or bad thing to do. Encourage them to come up with items in both columns. Review as a group.

VI. Activities Assignment

The activities that follow involve picking a current interpersonal problem and using the worksheets to problem-solve. Spend a few minutes with group members individually, selecting interpersonal problems. If they can't think of problems, select ones that they have worked on in group session before or ones that have given them difficulty with compliance. Also select additional topics from the fear hierarchy (Group Session 5, Section III) for real life exposure. Be sure to work with each group member to work out the details of the assignment.

1. Complete the "Problem-Solving Practice" worksheet.

2. Continue with real life exposure (using the "Problem-Solving Assignment" worksheet).

PROBLEM-SOLVING PRACTICE

Name: _____

In the box, write about a problem that you are having. Then complete the rest of the page.

What is the problem that you will work on?

Negative Thoughts About Problem	**Hot Seat Thoughts**
_____	_____
_____	_____
_____	_____
_____	_____

Possible Things You Could Do About It:

_____
_____
_____
_____
_____
_____
_____
_____
_____

Which one is best? Think about the pluses and minuses, or pros and cons, of each, and put a ** next to the one you want to try first.

Try it! How did it work?

PROBLEM-SOLVING ASSIGNMENT

Name: _____

This week, I am going to:

1) _____

This shows you how I felt when I did it:

	When / Where?	Fear Thermometer Rating		
		Before	After	Highest
1st time				
2nd time				
3rd time				
4th time				
5th time				

2) _____

This shows you how I felt when I did it:

	When / Where?	Fear Thermometer Rating		
		Before	After	Highest
1st time				
2nd time				
3rd time				
4th time				
5th time				

PRACTICE WITH SOCIAL PROBLEM-SOLVING

I. Activities Review

Review the problem-solving assignment. Review obstacles to problem-solving practice, and ask the group to generate new ideas for how to handle it if a group member is stuck. Some group members will not be able to overcome problems because of the nature of the problem. When this happens, point out that the group members made their best efforts but that not everything is under their control. Point out that they CAN control how they think and act, and, therefore, how to feel about the problem. Help group members find ways to feel better about the situations, using Hot Seat exercises or suggesting relaxation, if appropriate.

Review real life exposure practice and determine if continued work is necessary. If so, address this individually via parent phone calls or private discussions with the children. If children are reporting low Fear Thermometer levels for most things on their lists, congratulate them and address the need to continue.

II. Practice with Problem-Solving and Hot Seat

In this part of the session, most of the time is devoted to practice and review. Depending on the group, time can be devoted to problem-solving, to the Hot Seat, or, in most cases, to both. Focus the group and individual members on real life problems that are currently interfering with their lives. Use this

AGENDA	I. Activity Review II. Practice with Problem-Solving and Hot Seat III. Review of Key Concepts (No Activities Assignment)

OBJECTIVES

1. Build skills: Challenging negative thoughts.
2. Build skills: Social problem-solving.
3. Help children deal with real life problems.

SPECIAL SUPPLIES

time to consolidate techniques and help children develop skills to handle real problems.

Group Activity:

Divide the group into two teams. Present a problem that has several people involved (see the example that follows, but try to use something relevant to the group). Assign the role of Joe to one team and the role of Anna to the other. First, use the Hot Seat to challenge negative thoughts for each of the roles. Then, have each group follow the problem-solving steps to make a decision on what to do for each role. Compare decisions and discuss as a group.

Example:

Joe, Anna, and Dana are all meeting at the school dance on Friday night. They have been friends since elementary school. Right after they get to the dance, Joe and Dana want to leave to get something to eat. Anna wants to stay at the dance—there is a boy that she likes there. They tell her to stay, but she says she wants them to stay too. They still want to leave.

Assign the thoughts of Joe to one group, the thoughts of Anna to the other. Have each team do the Hot Seat to counteract negative thoughts leading to anger for Joe/Anna and then brainstorm solutions, weigh pros and cons, and pick a solution. Convene the two teams and ask them to present the solution and reason they picked it. If the solutions match (work for both parties), it is the end of the exercise. If they do not match, have them negotiate a compromise that works for both teams.

III. Review of Key Concepts

Structure an informal review of the key concepts the children have learned. One option is to create a trivia game and to give points for correct answers. Examples of questions:

"Name three common reactions to trauma."

"What is one question you can ask yourself when you have a negative thought?"

"Name another way (besides asking yourself questions) to combat negative thoughts."

"What is a good thing to do if you aren't sure how to handle a problem?"

"When something bad happens to us, is it better to think about it and talk about it, or to try to avoid it completely?"

RELAPSE PREVENTION AND GRADUATION

I. Relapse Prevention

The goal of this part of the session is to consolidate skills and anticipate future problems of group members. Use this time to help group members summarize their experiences in the program. Work on relapse prevention by anticipating future problems and how the children will handle them. Make sure to highlight group members' strengths as well as areas in which they should continue to practice skills.

"Since this is your last group, let's take a few minutes to review with you how it went and what you'll do in the future. Let's talk about:

1. *What you got out of the group.*

2. *What you see as the biggest challenges you'll face in the next few months or few years.*

3. *How you can apply the skills you learned here to tackle those challenges."*

Highlight avoidance as problematic, and make the following point:

"Avoidance can easily creep back into your life. You'll notice that you've stopped thinking about the event, talking about it, going certain places, doing certain things [use examples from group]. If that happens, use the skills you learned here to start doing all those things again, until it gets easy.

4. *How you can recognize avoidance. What are the warning signs? What can you do?"*

Spend a few minutes discussing any future contact you will have with the group, if any (e.g., reunions, booster sessions, individual

contact). Tell them how to reach you (if applicable) or how to get additional help somewhere else if they need it.

> **Parent phone call:**
>
> If you plan to make parent phone calls at the end of group, remind group members that this will occur. Use the phone call to review the group member's progress and areas that require additional work. Highlight progress and strengths to parents. Make any referrals or plans necessary to continue treatment with the parent and group member together.

II. Graduation Ceremony

The purpose of this part of the session is to provide closure to the group. If possible, present the group with certificates of completion, bring in food and beverages, or give little gifts to the group members to acknowledge their accomplishments in the group. Summarize the main accomplishment for each group member in some fashion or other, and highlight strengths.

Examples:

"When Pavlos started group, it was really hard for him to talk about what happened. In the group, he was able to draw pictures, and now he can probably talk about it to whomever he wants."

"Cindy has been working hard on the problems with her sister. Now she knows how she wants to handle it."

Parent Education Program

I. Introductions and Agenda

Introduce yourself and the role you have in the program. Briefly describe what the purpose and agenda are for these two sessions:

*"**Session 1** is to tell you a little bit about how children react to stress, to explain the framework we'll use in the group your children are in, and to teach you a way to help your children relax.*

*"**Session 2** is to help you learn new ways to help your children feel less afraid or nervous."*

II. Education About Common Reactions to Trauma

This part of the session conveys information about general types of problems that children experience when they have been exposed to traumatic life events. The goal is to normalize symptoms. Explain that the children will learn about these reactions but that it is really important for parents to understand them too. If parents understand the many problems that can result from traumatic experiences, they might be more understanding and supportive of the children, and less frustrated or worried about them.

Depending on the size of the group, this part of the session can be run as a lecture or as a discussion. Write the main points on a board or overhead transparency, and distribute copies of the "Handout for Parents" so that parents can make notes on it if they wish.

Make the following points during the presentation:

AGENDA

I. Introductions and Agenda

II. Education About Common Reactions to Trauma

III. Explanation of *CBITS*

IV. Teaching Your Child to Measure Fear

V. How to Help Your Child Relax

VI. Wrap-Up

OBJECTIVES

1. Reduce stigma around trauma exposure and reactions.
2. Lay groundwork for improving parent-child communication.

❑ All of the problems listed are common reactions to severe stress.

❑ The group for the children is designed to help with these specific problems.

❑ Parents may notice that they have some of these same problems because of stressful things they themselves have gone through.

Common Reactions to Stress or Trauma

Having nightmares or trouble sleeping. When something really scary or upsetting happens, it takes awhile to figure out exactly what happened and what it means. After severe stress or trauma, people tend to keep thinking about what happened in order to "digest" it, just like your stomach has to work to digest a big meal. This can take a long time. Nightmares are one way of digesting what happened to you.

Thinking about it all the time. This is another way to digest what happened. Just like having nightmares, thinking about the trauma all the time is a problem because it makes you feel upset. It can be unpleasant.

Wanting to NOT think or talk about it. This is natural, since it is upsetting to think about a past stress or trauma, and it can make you feel all sorts of emotions. Avoiding it makes things easier, but only for a little while. It's important to digest what happened sooner or later. So, while avoiding it sometimes makes sense, you have to set aside some time to digest it also. This group can be the time and place you set aside to digest what happened to you.

Avoiding places, people, or things that make you think about it. Just like not wanting to talk about or think about the trauma, avoiding situations that remind you of what happened can help you feel better right then. The problem with this, though, is that it keeps you from doing normal things that are an important part of your life. The goal of this group is to get you back to the point where you are able to do whatever you want to do, without worrying about whether it will remind you of what happened.

Feeling scared for no reason. Sometimes this happens because you remember what happened to you, or you are thinking about what happened. Other times it happens because your body is so tense all the time that you just start feeling scared. Either way, we can work on helping you feel calmer when it happens.

Feeling "crazy" or out of control. If all of these things are problems for you, you can start to feel really out of control or even crazy. Don't worry, though; these problems don't mean that you are going crazy. They are all normal reactions to stress or trauma, and there are ways to help you feel better.

Not being able to remember parts of what happened. This happens to a lot of people.

The stressful event can be so awful that your memory doesn't work the way it usually does. Sometimes it gets easier to remember later on, and sometimes it gets harder. This can be frustrating, but it is really normal.

Having trouble concentrating at school or at home. With all the nervousness you are feeling and all the time you are spending thinking about what happened, it can be hard to concentrate on school work or even on what your friends or family say to you.

Being on guard to protect yourself; feeling like something bad is about to happen. After something bad happens to you, it makes sense to be prepared for another bad thing to happen. The problem with this is that you can spend so much time waiting for the next bad thing to happen that you don't have time or energy for other things in your life. Also, it is scary to think something bad is going to happen.

Jumping when there is a loud noise. This is one way that your body says it is prepared for action, in case something else happens. As you begin to feel calmer, this will go away.

Feeling anger. Some people feel angry about the stress or trauma that happened, or about the things that happened afterward. Other people just feel angry all the time, at everything and everybody. Both of these are normal and will get better as you begin to digest what happened to you.

Feeling shame. Sometimes people are ashamed about what happened to them or how they acted. Even though it's hard to believe, this gets better the more that you talk about what happened. If you keep it a secret, it's hard for the shame to go away.

Feeling guilt. People can feel guilty about what happened or about something they did or did not do. Sometimes you blame yourself for things that you couldn't control. You may also feel guilty for upsetting your parents. Guilty feelings can make it hard to talk about what happened.

Feeling sadness/grief/loss. Sometimes stress events or traumas include losing someone close to you or losing something that is important to you. This makes you feel sad and down. We'll help you talk about these feelings in the group.

Feeling bad about yourself. Sometimes, all this stress can make you feel really bad about yourself, like you're a bad person or that no one likes you. This makes it harder to be friendly and to have fun with others.

Having physical health problems and complaints. Stress has an effect on your body as well. People sometimes get sick more often or notice pain and discomfort more often when they have been under stress.

III. Explanation of *CBITS*

This part of the session provides an overview of how thoughts and behaviors influence the feelings. Draw a triangle on the board. Write the phrase "Stress or Trauma" to one side, with an arrow pointing at the triangle. See **Figure 2**.

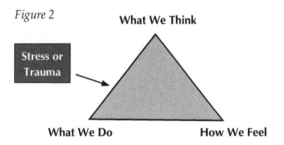

Figure 2

What We Think

Stress or Trauma

What We Do   How We Feel

Start by defining stress, soliciting examples from the group. Try to get a mixture of traumatic events (violence, accidents) and stress (immigration, leaving others behind, living in poverty).

"What do I mean by stress or trauma? Can you give some examples of things that might happen to a child that are stressful?" [Elicit ideas about stressful events, and list under the "Stress or Trauma" line.]

"When something stressful happens [use one of their examples], *how does that change what you think? What you do? What you feel?"*

Make the point that stress or trauma causes all of these to change and that each then impacts the others, making you feel worse. A possible example:

"Your children are in a car accident. That's the stress or trauma. Afterwards, they feel shaky, nervous, upset. They think that riding in a car is really dangerous, and they don't want to go in a car again. When you ask if they want to go shopping with you, they say no and stay home because they don't want to be in the car."

Explain how the program is going to help with things like this:

"Your children are all in this program because they had something really stressful happen to them. In this program, we are going to work on all three corners of the triangle. We are going to:

- *Teach the children some exercises that will make them FEEL better and less nervous or upset.*

- *Teach them some ways to THINK about things that will also make them feel better.*

- *Teach the children some ways to DO things so that they are able to do everything you want them to be able to do, without feeling upset when they do them."*

Explain the importance of practice and that activities will be assigned:

"One very important part of this program is PRACTICE. Learning new skills in this program is like learning to ride a bicycle or to

drive a car. At first, the skills feel uncomfortable, and it is hard to figure out how to do them. But if you practice the skills over and over again, eventually it becomes so easy and natural that you don't even have to think about it—you can ride the bike without thinking about balancing the bike and steering it and putting on the brakes when you need them. We will be practicing the new skills in the group and also asking your children to practice certain things at home between groups. The more that you can support and encourage the children to practice, the faster they will learn to use these skills to handle stress."

IV. Teaching Your Child to Measure Fear

Briefly introduce the idea of the Fear Thermometer so that parents will understand what it is and how their children will use it (see Appendix B).

"Part of what we'll be teaching your children is how to talk about how nervous or afraid they are. We will do this by teaching them to use a "Fear Thermometer." Like a thermometer that measures temperature, the Fear Thermometer measures how scared or upset the children feel."

Show the Fear Thermometers that indicate varying amounts of distress, and make sure that parents understand it. Use a personal example given by someone in the group to show how people feel at different times. Explain that the "10" on the Fear Thermometer is kept for those times when you are completely and utterly scared and upset.

V. How to Help Your Child Relax

The goal of this part of the session is to train parents in progressive muscle relaxation and relaxed breathing. Present the following rationale:

"Stress makes our bodies tense, and feeling nervous or upset makes it even worse. But there are ways to relax your body that will make you feel calmer. We are going to be teaching your children one way to relax, and we want to teach it to you also. That way, when your children have trouble sleeping or are feeling very worried, you can use it to help them relax."

Ask parents to lean back in their chairs, close their eyes, and follow your instructions.

"I'd like you to start by thinking of a place that makes you really comfortable, like your bed, or the bathtub, or the couch, or the beach. Imagine that you are lying down there or sitting comfortably. Take a breath in [wait three to four seconds] and out [wait three to four seconds], in . . . and out . . . in . . . and out. . . . Try to keep breathing this way as we continue. And keep thinking about your most comfortable spot.

"Now I'd like you to make a fist, and squeeze it really tight. You can open your eyes and see how I'm doing it if you're not sure how. Hold it. Now relax it completely; shake it out. Do it again—make a fist. Now relax it completely. Can you feel the difference between how it was when it was tight and now how it feels when it's relaxed? Let's do the same thing for the rest of your arm. Tighten up your whole arm, like you are making a muscle, and hold it. Now relax it completely. Do it again. Tighten, now relax. Now let's move to your shoulders. Bring your shoulders up to your ears and tighten them, hold it. Now relax. Do that again. Bring your shoulders way up near your ears, hold it, now relax them completely. Make sure your hands, arms, and shoulders are completely relaxed. Breathe in . . . and out . . . in . . . and out.

"Let's work on your face now. Scrunch up your face as tight as you can, close your eyes tight, scrunch up your mouth, and hold it. Now relax. Try that again. Tighten up your whole face, and hold it. Now relax it. Keep breathing like we did before . . . in . . . and out . . . in . . . and out.

"Next comes your body. Arch your back as much as you can, put your shoulders way back, like I am doing. Hold it. Now relax that. Next, lean forward onto your knees and curl your back the other way, and tighten up your stomach as much as you can. Hold it. Now relax it. Do that again, hold it, and relax it. Keep breathing in . . . and out . . . in . . . and out.

"Let's work on your legs and feet. Straighten your legs up in the air in front of you, and bring your toes as close to your face as you can. Tighten up your bottom also. Now hold it. Relax. Do that again, hold it, and now relax. Next, point your toes as far as you can away from your face, and again tighten up your leg muscles. Hold it. Now relax. Do that again, hold it, and relax. Breathe in . . . and out . . . in . . . and out.*

"Think about all the parts of your body, and relax any part that is tight now. Let all the tension go out of your body. Breathe in . . . and out . . . in . . . and out. Now begin to open your eyes, sit back up, and be a part of the group again."

VI. Wrap-Up

Thank parents for coming and encourage them to attend Parent Session 2.

COMMON REACTIONS TO STRESS OR TRAUMA

There are many different ways that young people react to stressful life events. Below we've listed several kinds of reactions, all of which are very common. We've asked your child to show this list to you and to talk with you about which ones he or she has had problems with recently. You might also notice the way that you've reacted to stressful events in your own life. Feel free to call us if you have any questions about these problems or the way in which the group will address them.

Having nightmares or trouble sleeping. When something really scary or upsetting happens, it takes awhile to figure out exactly what happened and what it means. After severe stress or trauma, people tend to keep thinking about what happened in order to "digest" it, just like your stomach has to work to digest a big meal. Nightmares are one way of digesting what happened.

Thinking about it all the time. This is another way to digest what happened. Just like nightmares, thinking about the trauma all the time is a problem because it makes you feel upset. It can be unpleasant.

Wanting to NOT think or talk about it. This is natural, since it is upsetting to think about a past stress or trauma, and it can make you feel all sorts of emotions. Avoiding it makes things easier, but only for a little while. It's important to digest what happened sooner or later. So, while avoiding it sometimes makes sense, you have to set aside some time to digest it also.

Avoiding places, people, or things that make you think about it. Just like not wanting to talk about or think about the trauma, avoiding situations that remind you of what happened can help you feel better right then. The problem with this, though, is that it keeps you from do-ing normal things that are an important part of your life.

Feeling scared for no reason. Sometimes this happens because you remember what happened to you, or you are thinking about what happened. Other times it happens because your body is so tense all the time that you just start feeling scared.

Feeling "crazy" or out of control. If all of these things are problems for you, you can start to feel really out of control or even crazy. Don't worry, though; these problems don't mean that you are going crazy. They are all common reactions to stress or trauma.

Not being able to remember parts of what happened. This happens to a lot of people. The stressful event can be so awful that your memory doesn't work the way it usually does. Sometimes it gets easier to remember it later on, and sometimes it gets harder. This can be frustrating, but it's really normal.

Having trouble concentrating at school or at home. With all the nervousness you are feeling and all the time you are spending thinking about what happened, it can be hard to concentrate on school work or even what your friends or family say to you.

Being on guard to protect yourself; feeling like something bad is about to happen. After something bad happens to you, it makes sense to be prepared for another bad thing to happen. The problem with this is that you can spend so much time waiting for the next bad thing to happen that you don't have time or energy for other things in your life. Also, it is scary to think something bad is going to happen all the time.

Jumping when there is a loud noise. This is another way to say that your body is prepared for action, in case something else happens.

Feeling anger. Sometimes people feel angry about the stress or trauma that happened, or the things that happened afterward. Other times, people just feel angry all the time, at everything and everybody.

Feeling shame. Sometimes people are ashamed about what happened to them, or how they acted. Even though it's hard to believe, this gets better the more that you talk about what happened. If you keep it a secret, it's hard for the shame to go away.

Feeling guilt. People can feel guilty about what happened or about something they did or did not do. Sometimes you blame yourself for things that you couldn't control. You may also feel guilty for upsetting other people. Guilty feelings can make it hard to talk about what happened.

Feeling sadness/grief/loss. Sometimes stress events include losing someone close to you or losing something that is important to you. This makes you feel sad and down.

Feeling bad about yourself. Sometimes, all this stress can make you feel really bad about yourself, like you're a bad person or that no one likes you. This makes is harder to be friendly and to have fun with others.

Having physical health problems and complaints. Stress has an effect on your body as well. People tend to get sick more often and to notice pain and discomfort more often when they have been under stress.

I.   Introductions and Agenda

Introduce yourself and your role in the program for any parents who missed the first session. Briefly remind parents of what they learned last time and what you will cover this time:

*"**Session 1** is to tell you a little bit about how children react to stress, to explain the framework we'll use in the group your children are in, and to teach you a way to help your children relax."*

*"**Session 2** is to help you learn new ways to help your children feel less afraid or nervous."*

II.   Teaching Children to Look at Their Thoughts

The goal of this part of the session is to tell parents about the cognitive portion of the program. Begin by describing the way that stress can influence thinking:

"When children are under stress, they can have really negative ideas about themselves, about the world in general, or about why the stress happened. For example, after children immigrate to the U.S., they might think things like:

'My life will never be the same.'

'I'll never be happy again.'

'I will never fit in here in the U.S.'

"After children go through traumatic events, they often think that they are to blame in some way or that what happened is their fault. They also usually think bad things about themselves

AGENDA

I.	Introductions and Agenda
II.	Teaching Children to Look at Their Thoughts
III.	Teaching Children to Face Their Fears
IV.	Teaching Children to Digest What Happened to Them
V.	Teaching Children to Solve Everyday Problems
VI.	Wrap-Up

OBJECTIVES

1. Educate parents about techniques used in the program.
2. Enable parents to support children during program.

SPECIAL SUPPLIES

1. Copies of the Parent Handouts
2. Copies of the Fear Thermometers
3. Copies of one of the Activity worksheets from a group session

('I'm no good') and think that the world is more dangerous than it really is ('There is no place where I am safe' or 'I can't trust anyone').

"These kinds of thoughts make children feel even worse. Negative thoughts are often not completely true. For instance, it's probably not true that the children will never be happy again or that they can't trust anyone. When negative thoughts aren't true, they still make us upset unless we realize that they aren't true.

"We will be teaching the children to pay attention to the way they think about things. If they notice some negative thinking, we'll teach them some questions to ask themselves to make sure that they aren't thinking inaccurately.

"Some of the questions your children will start to ask themselves are:

Is there another way to look at this?

Is there another reason why this would happen?

What's the worst thing that can happen?

What's the best thing that can happen?

What is the most likely thing to happen?

Is there anything I can do about this?

What is the evidence that this thought is true?

Has something like this happened to me before?

Has this happened with other people?"

Using the "Examples of Thoughts" handout that follows, take a few minutes to go through some of the questions you've listed. Show how the questions might help people to realize that their thoughts are not accurate and that there are more accurate ways to look at the situations. Show parents the examples on the handout to indicate how the children will be taught to think more accurately.

Take a few minutes to discuss any concerns and answer any questions that parents have about the process.

III. Teaching Children to Face Their Fears

The goal of this part of the session is to teach parents about the real life exposures that the children will do in the group. Begin by explaining how avoidance builds up and interferes with recovery:

"One way that people deal with stress is to try to avoid it. You have probably all had the experience of NOT wanting to do something that will make you feel nervous or afraid. This usually works for a short time—we can sometimes avoid something that will be hard for us. But over time, it can interfere with your life. For instance, some

of you may feel nervous or anxious when you try to speak English. So, you might try to avoid speaking English unless you really have to. But this interferes with learning English, so it makes it harder to speak English for a longer period of time. The same thing happens with children who go through stressful experiences. They avoid the things that make them uncomfortable. They begin to avoid more and more often. For instance, children who feel afraid of school will sometimes skip school, but that just makes it harder to go back to school again.

"In the group, we will be teaching your children to face their fears. What do we mean by facing your fears? We mean trying to do something that you are afraid of over and over again until it becomes normal and easy. [Give an example, such as: "I used to be nervous speaking in front of groups of people, but the more I did it, the easier it got. Now I just get a little bit nervous, but I know I can do it without having any problems." {Pass out copies of the "Facing Your Fears" handout.]

"With the children, we will start by making a list of situations that make each of them feel anxious or upset and then rank the situations in terms of how much anxiety each situation causes (using the Fear Thermometer). We will be careful about a couple of things when we do this:

1. *The situations on the list must be SAFE. We will not include situations that involve being exposed to violence in person, doing anything dangerous, or being in unsafe environments (e.g., out alone in a deserted area at night).*

2. *Some situations are designed to make people feel nervous or excited, and are hard to work on. These include watching scary movies, riding roller coasters, etc. We will not work on these kinds of situations either.*

"We will concentrate instead on the answers to the following questions:

- *Are there any things that you used to do regularly that you stopped doing after the stress or trauma you went through? Examples: going to places that remind you of what happened, doing things that you were doing when the stress or trauma happened.*

- *Have you started avoiding things like being alone in certain places, being in the dark, sleeping by yourself?*

- *Do you avoid talking to people about what happened? Is there anyone that you'd like to be able to talk to about it?*

- *Do you avoid reading things or watching certain TV programs that remind you about what happened?*

- *Do you avoid certain objects that make you nervous or upset because they were there when it happened?*

"Then children will rate each situation using the Fear Thermometer [show it again], *and they will participate in activities.* [Describe the typical kind of assignments and read through a sample Activity Worksheet from one of the group sessions.]

"You can help by working with your children to do the assignments. Sometimes your children will need to do something with you first, before being able to do it alone. We also need you to help your children face their fears by facing your own. You might notice that you are nervous about doing certain things too, because of the kinds of stressors you have faced. By helping your children, you may find that you become more comfortable with doing these things.

Take a few minutes to discuss any concerns and answer any questions that parents have about the process.

IV. Teaching Children to Digest What Happened to Them

The goal of this part of the session is to prepare parents for the trauma-focused work that their children will do in the group.

"We are going to work with your children on the stresses or traumas that they have gone through.

"Have you ever eaten too much all at once and felt really full and sick afterwards? And you wish you never ate that much? Your stomach feels sick because it's got too much in it at once. That food feels like its filling up your whole body. Your stomach has more than it can handle.

"The way you think about the stressful event you went through can also feel like that—it's too much to digest at once, so it bothers you a lot. Just like with the meal, you need to "digest" it sooner or later though. Even though the stress probably seems really overwhelming when you think about it now, eventually, with enough work, you can make it smaller. We're going to help your children digest what happened.

"By thinking about the stress or trauma where it is safe (with a counselor or in the group), a couple of things will happen:

1. *Over time, if your children work on digesting the stresses or traumas, they will feel less upset each time they think about it. By the end of group sessions, your children will be able to think about what happened and feel OK.*

2. *Your children will learn that thinking about the stresses or traumas won't make them flip out or go crazy—that it's a bad memory and it can't hurt them anymore.*

3. *Your children will learn that they can take control of the way they feel and do something to make themselves feel better.*

"We will work on the traumas by asking your children to imagine them or to draw pictures of them or to talk about them in the group sessions."

Take a few minutes to discuss any concerns and answer any questions that parents have about the process.

III. Teaching Children to Solve Everyday Problems

The purpose of this part of the session is to briefly introduce the idea that solving problems with other people takes practice and to explain how this process will work in the group. Begin by getting examples from parents of the kinds of problems that their children face. If they do not volunteer any, supply some of the following:

❑ Getting in arguments with friends.

❑ Disagreeing with parents about rules at home.

❑ Disagreeing with brothers and sisters.

❑ Having trouble in a class at school.

Explain that the group will work on the following parts of the problems:

❑ Looking at the thoughts the children have about the problems, to make sure they are seeing problems accurately.

❑ Coming up with a list of possible solutions about how to handle the problems.

❑ Looking at the possible solutions to see the positives and negatives of each one.

❑ Trying out solutions to see if they work.

Take a few minutes to discuss any concerns and answer any questions that parents have about the process.

IV. Wrap-Up

Take a few minutes to praise the parents on taking time to attend the meeting(s), and remind them of how to reach you as the program continues:

"I want to thank you all for coming tonight. I know it takes a lot of effort to get here on a school night, and it really shows your love and concern for your children. I hope you've gotten a better idea of what this program is all about, and I want you to know that you can call me with any questions or concerns at any time."

EXAMPLES OF THOUGHTS

Negative Thoughts	Hot Seat Thoughts
If I fall asleep, I'll have nightmares.	• I don't have nightmares every night, so I might not have them tonight. • Nightmares aren't real, they can't hurt me. • I need to get some sleep for school tomorrow, even if it means I have nightmares.
If I fall asleep, something bad will happen.	• I'm safe in my house and my bed. My family is here to protect me. • If something bad happens, I'll wake up and be able to deal with it then.
Lying down in my bed makes me feel nervous.	• I can practice my relaxation if I feel nervous. • I can remind myself that I am safe. • It's OK to feel nervous for a little while; eventually I'll fall asleep.

FACING YOUR FEARS

1) Choose something from the list that you are sure you can manage, with a rating of no more than 4 on the Fear Thermometer for your first try.

2) Figure out when and where you can try to do the thing you chose.
    – You need to do it over and over again, not just once or twice.
    – You need to be able to do it SAFELY:
        • Don't do anything that will put you in danger.
        • Don't do anything without telling someone first.

3) Tell a parent what you are going to do. Make sure your parent understands what you plan and can help you with it, if you need help.

4) When you do it, stick with it no matter how nervous you feel. Keep at it until you begin to feel a little bit less nervous or upset. You can use your relaxation technique if you need it. You might need to stick with it for a long time, up to an hour, before you start to feel better. If you don't feel better after an hour, make sure to try it again and again. Eventually, with enough practice, you'll start to feel more comfortable.

5) Fill out the activities form to show how you felt on the Fear Thermometer before and after each time you did it. Also, tell what your highest level on the Fear Thermometer was. Talk to your group leader if you don't see any improvement.

Teacher Education
Program

TEACHER EDUCATION SESSION

I. Introductions and Agenda

Introduce yourself and the role you have in the program. Briefly describe what the purpose and agenda are for this session:

❑ To describe common reactions to trauma and provide a model for thinking about trauma.

❑ To describe elements of the *CBITS* program.

❑ To offer tips for teaching children who have been traumatized.

II. Education about Common Reactions to Trauma

This part of the session conveys information about general types of problems that children experience when they have been exposed to traumatic life events. If teachers understand that many problems can result from traumatic experiences, they might be more understanding and supportive of the children and less frustrated or worried about them. Highlight possible classroom manifestations of the problems, and lead a discussion about the way these problems are often attributed to other causes (e.g., ADHD).

Make the following points:

❑ All of the problems are common reactions to severe stress.

❑ The group for the children is designed to help with these specific problems.

❑ Children often have comorbid problems, like depression, disruptive behavior prob-

lems, or ADHD. You are not trying to suggest that trauma is the root cause of all the problems that the children have. Rather, trauma-related symptoms are part of the picture.

❑ Other problems, like ADHD and depression, can sometimes mask trauma-related symptoms. The reverse is also true—trauma-related symptoms can mask other severe problems. Diagnosis and treatment are complex because it is necessary to tease apart the problems in order to implement appropriate treatments.

Common Reactions to Stress or Trauma

People cope with trauma in different ways. You may find a student exhibiting one or more of the following symptoms:

Having nightmares or trouble sleeping. When something really scary or upsetting happens, it takes awhile to figure out exactly what happened and what it means. After severe stress or trauma, people tend to keep thinking about what happened in order to "digest" it, just like your stomach has to work to digest a big meal. This can take a long time. *Classroom manifestation: fatigue, sleepiness during the day.*

Thinking about it all the time/re-enacting it. This is another way to digest what happened. Just like having nightmares, thinking about the trauma all the time is a problem because it makes you feel upset. It can be unpleasant. *Classroom manifestation: trouble concentrating, tearfulness, repetitive play around theme of trauma.*

Wanting to NOT think or talk about it. This is natural, since it is upsetting to think about a past stress or trauma and can make you feel all sorts of emotions. Avoiding trauma memory makes things easier, but only for a little while. It's important to digest what happened sooner or later. So, while avoiding it sometimes makes sense, you have to set aside some time to digest it also. *Classroom manifestation: trouble sitting still, constantly creating distractions, not wanting to talk about problems.*

Avoiding places, people, or things that make you think about it. Just like not wanting to talk about or think about the trauma, avoiding situations that remind you of what happened can help you feel better right then. The problem with this, though, is that it keeps you from doing normal things that are an important part of your life. *Classroom manifestation: resistance to doing certain things or going certain places, without a clear explanation of why; absenteeism because of avoidance of things on the way to school or of school itself.*

Feeling scared for no reason. Sometimes this happens because you remember what happened to you, or you are thinking about what happened. Other times it happens because your body is so tense all the time that you just start feeling scared. *Classroom manifestation: getting upset easily.*

Feeling "crazy" or out of control. If all of these things are problems for you, you can start to feel really out of control or even crazy. Don't worry, though; these problems don't mean that you are going crazy. They are all normal reactions to stress or trauma. *Classroom manifestation: getting upset easily.*

Not being able to remember parts of what happened. This happens to a lot of people. The stressful event can be so awful that your memory doesn't work the way it usually does. Sometimes it gets easier to remember later on, and sometimes it gets harder. This can be frustrating, but it is really normal. *No clear classroom manifestation.*

Having trouble concentrating at school or at home. With all the nervousness you are feeling and all the time you are spending thinking about what happened, it can be hard to concentrate on school work or even on what your friends or family say to you. *Classroom manifestation: concentration problems, not finishing activities, doing worse on school work and tests.*

Being on guard to protect yourself; feeling like something bad is about to happen. After something bad happens to you, it makes sense to be prepared for another bad thing to happen. The problem with this is that you can spend so much time waiting for the next bad thing to happen that you don't have time or energy for other things in your life. Also, it is scary to think something bad is going to happen. *Classroom manifestation: wanting to face the door or have back to wall, keeping alert at all times.*

Jumping when there is a loud noise. This is one way that your body says it is prepared for action, in case something else happens. *Classroom manifestation: being startled easily.*

Feeling anger. Some people feel angry about the stress or trauma that happened, or about the things that happened afterward. Other people just feel angry all the time, at everything and everybody. *Classroom manifestation: increased fights with peers, being oppositional.*

Feeling shame. Sometimes people are ashamed about what happened to them or how they acted. Even though it's hard to believe, this gets better the more that you talk about what happened. If you keep it a secret, it's hard for the shame to go away. *Classroom manifestation: withdrawal from peers, poor eye-contact, negative self-statements.*

Feeling guilt. People can feel guilty about what happened or about something they did or did not do. Sometimes you blame yourself for things that you couldn't control. You may also feel guilty for upsetting your parents. Guilty feelings can make it hard to talk about what happened. *Classroom manifestation: negative self-statements.*

Feeling sadness/grief/loss. Sometimes stress events or traumas include losing someone close to you or losing something that is important to you. This makes you feel sad and down. *Classroom manifestation: tearfulness, clinging to parents or teachers, withdrawal from peers.*

Feeling bad about yourself. Sometimes all this can make you feel really bad about yourself, like you're a bad person or that no one likes you. This makes it harder to be friendly and to have fun with others. *Classroom manifestation: withdrawal from peers, negative self-statements.*

Having physical health problems and complaints. Stress has an effect on your body as well. People sometimes get sick more often or notice pain and discomfort more often when they have been under stress. *Classroom manifestation: more trips to the school nurse, absenteeism, complaints about stomachaches or headaches.*

III. Explanation of *CBITS*

This part of the session provides an overview of how thoughts and behaviors influence the feelings. Draw a triangle on the board. Write the phrase "Stress or Trauma" to one side, with an arrow pointing at the triangle. See **Figure 3**.

Figure 3

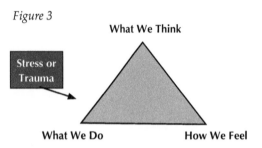

Start by defining stress, soliciting examples from the group. Try to get a mixture of traumatic events (violence, accidents) and stress (immigration, leaving others behind, living in poverty).

"What do I mean by stress or trauma? Can you give some examples of things that might happen to a child that are stressful?" [Elicit ideas about stressful events, and list under the "Stress or Trauma" line.]

"When something stressful happens [use one of their examples], *how does that change what you think? What you do? What you feel?"*

Make the point that stress or trauma causes all of these to change and that each then impacts the others, making you feel worse. A possible example:

"Marisol is in a car accident. That's the stress or trauma. Afterwards, she feels shaky, nervous, upset. She thinks that riding in a car is really dangerous, and she doesn't want to go in the car again. When her mother asks if she wants to go shopping with her, she says no and stays home, because she doesn't want to be in the car."

Explain how the program is going to help with things like this:

"In this program, we are going to work on all three corners of the triangle. We are going to:

- *Teach the children some exercises that will make them FEEL better and less nervous or upset.*

- *Teach them some ways to THINK about things that will also make them feel better.*

- *Teach the children some ways to DO things so that they are able to do everything they want to do without feeling upset when they do them."*

IV. Elements of the *CBITS* Program

Describe the elements of the *CBITS* program and the reasons for them:

❏ Relaxation exercises to combat anxiety.

❏ Education about common symptoms to normalize them.

❏ Work on negative, maladaptive thoughts to teach children to generate more positive, accurate, and flexible ways of interpreting problems. This is intended to combat negative ideas that the world is very dangerous or that the self is bad.

❏ Social problem-solving to help children cope with problems with friends and family members. This includes thinking about the problem, brainstorming possible solutions, and evaluating pros and cons of potential solutions.

❏ Real life exposure to trauma-related events and situations. This is used to combat trauma-related anxiety by gradual and repetitive exposure to trauma reminders and triggers of anxiety while being safe. Situations include things that were actually present during the trauma as well as things like being alone, sleeping alone, feeling vulnerable.

❏ Exposure to trauma memory in imagination or through drawing or telling others in the group. This is used to process the trauma and reduce anxiety related to thinking about or remembering the trauma.

V. Tips for Teaching Children Who Have Been Traumatized

The goal of this part of the session is to offer suggestions for dealing with children who have undergone trauma. Treat the teachers as experts and guide a discussion of ways in which they might help the children, covering all the following points:

❏ See children's behavior through a "trauma lens." This means taking into account the children's traumatic life events and trying to understand why they might be acting out. Try to remember that even the most disruptive behaviors can be driven by the fear and anxiety created during trauma exposure.

❏ Give children choices and consistency. Often traumatic events involve loss of control and/or chaos, so you can help children feel safe by providing them with some control and a sense of consistency.

❏ Understand that attempts by children to replay trauma through play or through their interactions with others is a way to cope with trauma. Resist their efforts to draw you into a repetition of the trauma. For instance, some children will provoke teachers in order to replay abusive situations at home.

❏ Understand that children who have experienced trauma have idiosyncratic triggers that make them highly anxious. Triggers may include many kinds of situations. If you are able to identify what they are, you can help the children by preparing them for the situation and making sure that they feel comfortable. For instance, children who don't like being alone may not want to go to the bathroom alone at school. Consider sending children to the bathrooms in pairs if this is a problem for a child in your classroom. It can also be helpful to warn children if you will be doing something out of the ordinary, such as turning off the lights or making a sudden loud noise.

❑ Seek support and consultation to prevent burn-out. Be aware that you can develop symptoms through "vicarious traumatization" or exposure to traumas through the children you work with.

VI. Answering Questions

Teachers often have questions about implementation. For example, they might ask, "Can I refer children to the group? Will I know who participates? What if the program conflicts with the timing of a test?" Be prepared to respond to these questions with the details of how *CBITS* will be implemented in your school.

Some teachers ask questions about specific children who are participating in the program. Be clear about how confidentiality of group participation and group content will be handled. In most school settings it is not possible to protect confidentiality about participation itself, though it is still possible (and important) to keep the content of group participation private and confidential. Thus, it is usually not appropriate to answer questions about content.

Other questions from teachers often center on specific traumatic incidents that have affected them or their schools. These questions or comments can be turned into discussion points and provide an opportunity to reiterate the common reactions to trauma.

Common Reactions to Stress or Trauma

There are many different ways that young people react to stressful life events. Below we've listed several kinds of reactions, all of which are very common. We've asked your child to show this list to you and to talk with you about which ones he or she has had problems with recently. You might also notice the way that you've reacted to stressful events in your own life. Feel free to call us if you have any questions about these problems or the way in which the group will address them.

Having nightmares or trouble sleeping. When something really scary or upsetting happens, it takes awhile to figure out exactly what happened and what it means. After severe stress or trauma, people tend to keep thinking about what happened in order to "digest" it, just like your stomach has to work to digest a big meal. Nightmares are one way of digesting what happened.

Thinking about it all the time. This is another way to digest what happened. Just like nightmares, thinking about the trauma all the time is a problem because it makes you feel upset. It can be unpleasant.

Wanting to NOT think or talk about it. This is natural, since it is upsetting to think about a past stress or trauma, and it can make you feel all sorts of emotions. Avoiding it makes things easier, but only for a little while. It's important to digest what happened sooner or later. So, while avoiding it sometimes makes sense, you have to set aside some time to digest it also.

Avoiding places, people, or things that make you think about it. Just like not wanting to talk about or think about the trauma, avoiding situations that remind you of what happened can help you feel better right then. The problem with this, though, is that it keeps you from doing normal things that are an important part of your life.

Feeling scared for no reason. Sometimes this happens because you remember what happened to you, or you are thinking about what happened. Other times it happens because your body is so tense all the time that you just start feeling scared.

Feeling "crazy" or out of control. If all of these things are problems for you, you can start to feel really out of control or even crazy. Don't worry, though; these problems don't mean that you are going crazy. They are all common reactions to stress or trauma.

Not being able to remember parts of what happened. This happens to a lot of people. The stressful event can be so awful that your memory doesn't work the way it usually does. Sometimes it gets easier to remember it later on, and sometimes it gets harder. This can be frustrating, but it's really normal.

Having trouble concentrating at school or at home. With all the nervousness you are feeling and all the time you are spending thinking about what happened, it can be hard to concentrate on school work or even what your friends or family say to you.

Being on guard to protect yourself; feeling like something bad is about to happen. After something bad happens to you, it makes sense to be prepared for another bad thing to happen. The problem with this is that you can spend so much time waiting for the next bad thing to happen that you don't have time or energy for other things in your life. Also, it is scary to think something bad is going to happen all the time.

Jumping when there is a loud noise. This is another way to say that your body is prepared for action, in case something else happens.

Feeling anger. Sometimes people feel angry about the stress or trauma that happened, or the things that happened afterward. Other times, people just feel angry all the time, at everything and everybody.

Feeling shame. Sometimes people are ashamed about what happened to them, or how they acted. Even though it's hard to believe, this gets better the more that you talk about what happened. If you keep it a secret, it's hard for the shame to go away.

Feeling guilt. People can feel guilty about what happened or about something they did or did not do. Sometimes you blame yourself for things that you couldn't control. You may also feel guilty for upsetting other people. Guilty feelings can make it hard to talk about what happened.

Feeling sadness/grief/loss. Sometimes stress events include losing someone close to you or losing something that is important to you. This makes you feel sad and down.

Feeling bad about yourself. Sometimes, all this stress can make you feel really bad about yourself, like you're a bad person or that no one likes you. This makes is harder to be friendly and to have fun with others.

Having physical health problems and complaints. Stress has an effect on your body as well. People tend to get sick more often and to notice pain and discomfort more often when they have been under stress.

Appendix A

Case Formulation Worksheet

CASE SUMMARY

School _____   Child Name _____

Group _____   Group Leader _____

Child's Stated Goals	Parent's Stated Goals

Primary Symptoms	Emphasis in Intervention

Special Issues

Progress in Treatment/Changes in Plan

Appendix B

Fear Thermometers

Fear Thermometer 1

Name: _____

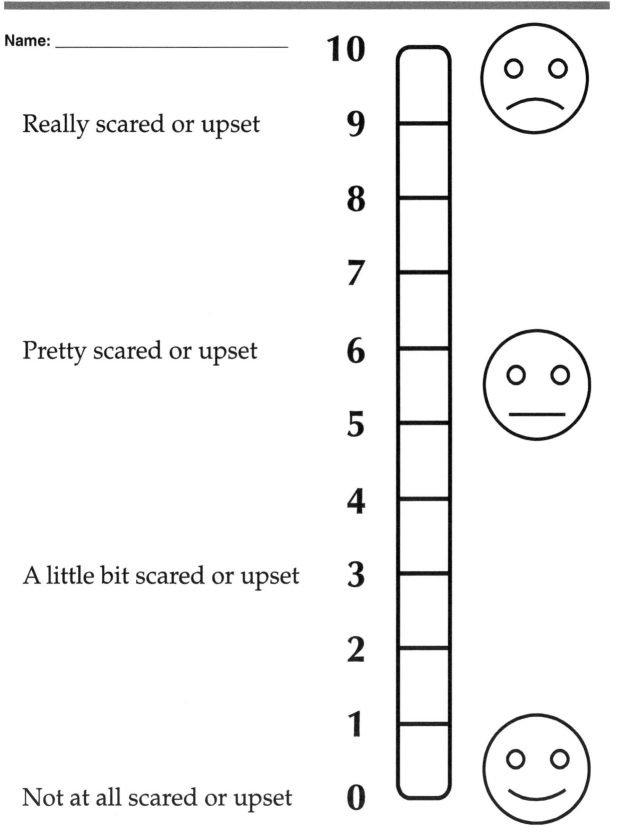

Really scared or upset — 10 9

8

7

Pretty scared or upset — 6

5

4

A little bit scared or upset — 3

2

1

Not at all scared or upset — 0

FEAR THERMOMETER 2

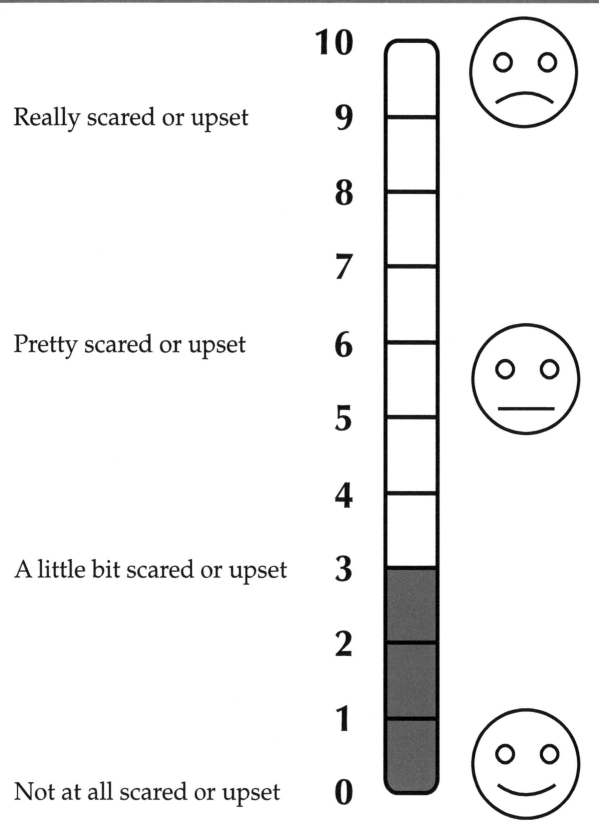

Really scared or upset

Pretty scared or upset

A little bit scared or upset

Not at all scared or upset

10
9
8
7
6
5
4
3
2
1
0

FEAR THERMOMETER 3

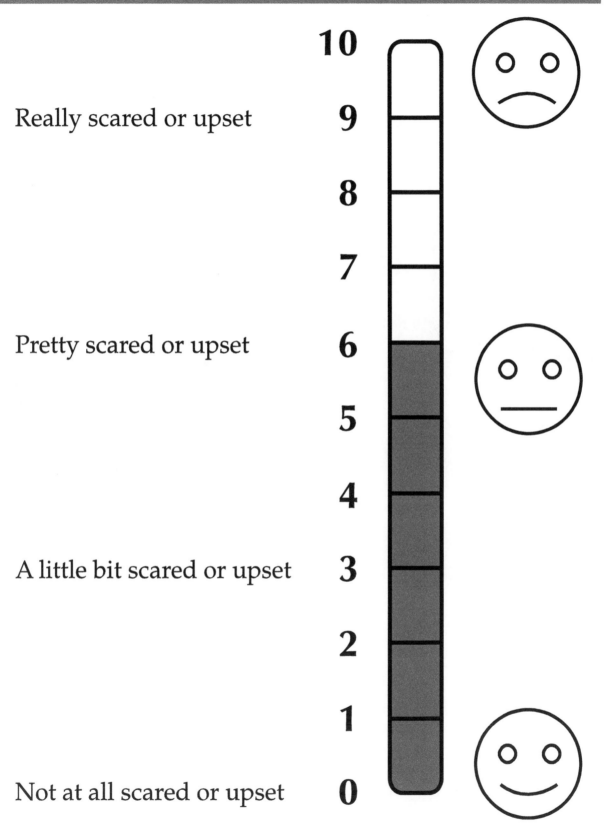

Really scared or upset

Pretty scared or upset

A little bit scared or upset

Not at all scared or upset

10
9
8
7
6
5
4
3
2
1
0

FEAR THERMOMETER 4

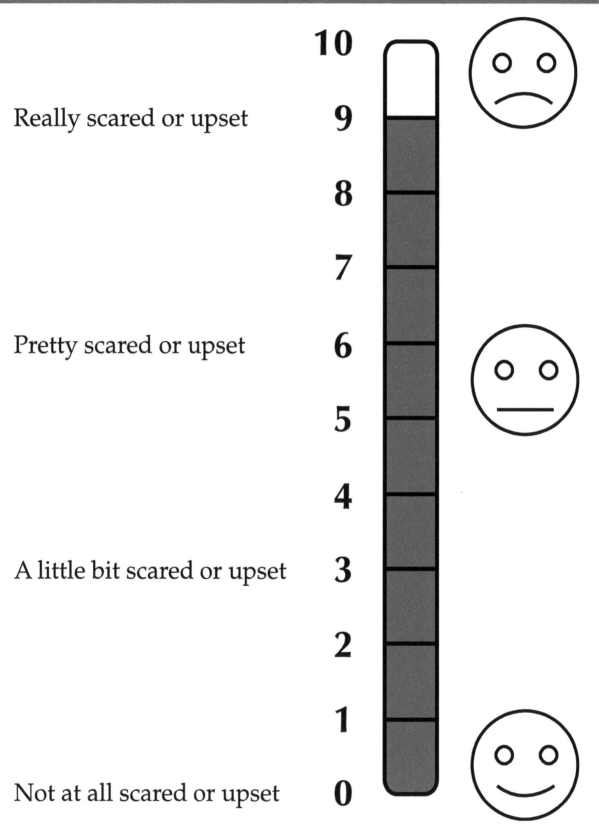

Really scared or upset

Pretty scared or upset

A little bit scared or upset

Not at all scared or upset

10
9
8
7
6
5
4
3
2
1
0

REFERENCES

Asarnow, J., Jaycox, L. H., Clarke, G., Lewinsohn, P., Hops, H., & Rohde, P. (1999a). *Stress and Your Mood: A Manual.* Los Angeles: UCLA School of Medicine.

Asarnow, J., Jaycox, L. H., Clarke, G., Lewinsohn, P., Hops, H., & Rohde, P. (1999b). *Stress and Your Mood: A Workbook.* Los Angeles: UCLA School of Medicine.

Bell, C. C., & Jenkins, E. J. (1991). Traumatic stress and children. *Journal of Health Care for the Poor & Underserved, 2*(1), 175–185.

Centers for Disease Control. (1990). Homicide among young black males—United States, 1978-1987. *Morbidity and Mortality Weekly Report, 37,* 543–545.

Cohen, J. A. (1998). *Practice parameters for the assessment and treatment of children and adolescents with posttraumatic stress disorder.* Washington, D.C.: American Academy of Child and Adolescent Psychiatry.

Delaney-Black, V., Covington, C., Ondersma, S. J., Nordstrom-Klee, B., Templin, T., Ager, J., Janisse, J., & Sokol, R. J. (2002). Violence exposure, trauma, and IQ and/or reading deficits among urban children. *Archives of Pediatrics & Adolescent Medicine, 156*(3), 280–285.

Farrell, A. D., & Bruce, S. E. (1997). Impact of exposure to community violence on violent behavior and emotional distress among urban adolescents. *Journal of Clinical Child Psychology, 26*(1), 2–14.

Finkelhor, D. (1995). The victimization of children: A developmental perspective. *American Journal of Orthopsychiatry, 65*(2). 177–193.

Finkelhor, D., & Dziuba-Leatherman, J. (1994). Children as victims of violence: A national survey. *Pediatrics, 94*(4 Pt. 1), 413–20.

Fitzpatrick, K. M., & Boldizar, J. P. (1993). The prevalence and consequences of exposure to violence among African American youth. *Journal of the American Academy of Child and Adolescent Psychiatry, 32*(2), 424–430.

Foa, E. B., Hearst, D. E., Dancu, C. V., Hembree, E., Jaycox, L. H., & Clark, D. M. (1994a). *Cognitive Restructuring and Prolonged Exposure Manual for Assault Victims.* Unpublished manual.

Foa, E. B., Hearst, D. E., Dancu, C. V., Hembree, E., & Jaycox, L. H. (1994b). *Prolonged Exposure Manual for Assault Victims.* Unpublished manual.

Foa, E. B., & Jaycox, L. H. (1999). Cognitive-behavioral treatment of post-traumatic stress disorder. In D. Spiegel (Ed.) *Efficacy and Cost-Effectiveness of Psychotherapy.* Washington, D.C.: American Psychiatric Press.

Foa, E. B., Treadwell, K., Johnson, K., & Feeny, N. C. (2001). The Child PTSD Symptom Scale: A preliminary examination of its psychometric properties. *Journal of Clinical Child Psychology, 30*(3), 376–384.

Garbarino, J., Dubrow, N., Kostelny, K., & Pardo, C. (1992). *Children in danger: Coping with the consequences of community violence.* San Francisco, CA: Jossey-Bass.

Gillham, J., Jaycox, L. H., Reivich, K. J., Seligman, M. E. P., & Silver, T. (1991). *Manual for Leaders of the Coping Skills Program for Children.* Unpublished manual. Copyright: Foresight, Inc.

Gillham, J., Reivich, K. J., Jaycox, L. H., & Seligman, M. E. P. (1995). Prevention of depressive symptoms in school children: Two-year follow-up. *Psychological Science, 6*(6), 343–351.

Grogger, J. (1997). Local violence and educational attainment. *The Journal of Human Resources, 32*(4), 659–682.

Hurt, H., Malmud, E., Brodsky, N. L., & Giannetta, J. (2001). Exposure to violence: Psychological and academic correlates in child witnesses. *Archives of Pediatrics & Adolescent Medicine, 155*(12), 1351–1356.

Jaycox, L. H., Reivich, K. J., Gillham, J., & Seligman, M. E. P. (1994). Prevention of depressive symptoms in school children. *Behaviour Research and Therapy, 32*(8), 801–816.

Jaycox, L. H., Stein, B., Kataoka, S., Wong, M., Fink, A., Escudera, P., & Zaragoza, C. (2002). Violence exposure, PTSD, and depressive symptoms among recent immigrant school children. *Journal of the American Academy of Child and Adolescent Psychiatry, 41*(9), 1104–1110.

Jenkins, E. J., & Bell, C. C. (1994). Post-traumatic stress disorder and violence among inner city high school students. In S. Friedman (Ed.), *Anxiety disorders in African Americans.* New York: Springer.

Kataoka, S., Stein, B. D., Jaycox, L. H., Wong, M., Escudero, P., Tu, W., Zaragoza, C., & Fink, A. (2003). A school-based mental health program for traumatized Latino immigrant children. *Journal of the American Academy of Child and Adolescent Psychiatry, 42*(3), 311–318.

Kilpatrick, D. G., Veronen, L. J., & Resick, P. A. (1982). Psychological sequelae to rape: Assessment and treatment strategies. In D. M. Dolays & R. L. Meredith (Eds.), *Behavioral medicine: Assessment and treatment strategies.* New York: Plenum Press, pp. 473–497.

Kliewer, W., Lopore, S. J., Oskin, D., & Johnson, P. D. (1998). The role of social and cognitive processes in children's adjustment to community violence. *Journal of Consulting & Clinical Psychology, 66*(1), 199–209.

Koop, C. E., & Lundberg, G. B. (1992). Violence in America: A public health emergency. Time to bite the bullet back. *Journal of the American Medical Association, 267*(22), 3075–3076.

Kovacs, M. (1981). Rating scales to assess depression in school-aged children. *Acta Paedopsychiatrica, 46*(5–6), 305–315.

Lewinsohn, P. M., Muñoz, R. F., Youngren, M. A., & Zeiss, A. M. (1986). *Control your depression.* New York: Prentice-Hall Press.

March, J. S., Amaya-Jackson, L., Murray, M. C., & Schulte, A. (1998). Cognitive-behavioral psychotherapy for children and adolescents with posttraumatic stress disorder after a single-incident stressor. *Journal of the American Academy of Child & Adolescent Psychiatry, 37*(6), 585–593.

Martinez, P., & Richters, J. E. (1993). The NIMH Community Violence Project: II. Children's distress symptoms associated with violence exposure. *Psychiatry Interpersonal and Biological Processes, 56*(1), 22–35.

Muñoz, R. F., & Miranda, J. (1986). *Group therapy manual for cognitive-behavioral treatment of depression.* San Francisco: San Francisco General Hospital, Depression Clinic.

Osofsky, J. D., Wewers, S., Hann, D. M., & Fick, A. C. (1993). Chronic community violence: What is happening to our children? *Psychiatry, 56*(1), 36–45.

Overstreet, S. (2000). Exposure to community violence: Defining the problem and understanding the consequences. *Journal of Child & Family Studies, 9*(1), 7–25.

Public Health Service (1990). *Healthy people 2000: National health promotion and disease prevention objectives.* Washington, D.C.: U.S .Department of Health and Human Services.

Putnam, F. W. (1997). *Dissociation in children and adolescents: A developmental perspective*. New York: Guilford Press.

Pynoos, R. S., Steinberg, A. M., & Goenjian, A. (1996). Traumatic stress in childhood and adolescence: Recent developments and current controversies. In B. A. van der Kolk, A. C. McFarlane, & L. Weisaeth (Eds.), *Traumatic stress: The effects of overwhelming experience on mind, body, and society* (pp. 331–358). New York: Guilford Press.

Richters, J. E., & Martinez, P. (1993) The NIMH Community Violence Project: I. Children as victims of and witnesses to violence. *Psychiatry Interpersonal and Biological Processes, 56*(1), 7–21.

Saigh, P. A., & Bremner, J. (Eds.) (1999). *Posttraumatic stress disorder: A comprehensive text*. Boston: Allyn & Bacon.

Saigh, P. A., Mroueh, M., & Bremner, J. D. (1997). Scholastic impairments among traumatized adolescents. *Behaviour Research & Therapy, 35*(5), 429–436.

Schwab-Stone, M. E., Ayers, T. S., Kasprow, W., Voyce, C., Barone, C., Shriver, T., & Weissberg, R. P. (1995). No safe haven: a study of violence exposure in an urban community. *Journal of the American Academy of Child & Adolescent Psychiatry, 34*(10), 1343–1352.

Singer, M. I., Anglin, T. M., Song, L. Y., & Lunghofer, L. (1995). Adolescents' exposure to violence and associated symptoms of psychological trauma. *Journal of the American Medical Association, 273*(6), 477–482.

Singer, M. I., Miller, D. B., Guo, S., Slovak, K., & Frierson, T. (1998). *The mental health consequences of children exposed to violence: Final report*. Cleveland, OH: Case Western Reserve University.

Stein, B. D., Jaycox, L. H., Kataoka, S. H., Wong, M., Tu, W., Elliot, M. N., & Fink, A. (2003). A mental health intervention for school children exposed to violence: A randomized controlled trial. *JAMA, 290*(5), 603–611.

Stein, B. D., Zima, B. T., Elliott, M. N., Burnan, M. A., Shahinfar, A., Fox, N. A., & Leavitt, L. A. (2001). Violence exposure among school-age children in foster care: Relationship to distress symptoms. *Journal of the American Academy of Child and Adolescent Psychiatry, 40*(5), 588–594.

Stein, B., Kataoka, S., Jaycox, L., Wong, M., Fink, A., Escudero, P., & Zaragoza, C. (2002). Theoretical basis and program design of a school-based mental health intervention for traumatized immigrant children: A collaborative research partnership. *Journal of Behavioral Health Services and Research, 29*(3), 318–326.